How To Get Awesome Results With Intermittent Fasting

Burn Fat, Lose Weight, Be Healthy

SECOND EDITION

LORI GEURIN

COPYRIGHT

READER RESULTS

"I'm down 25 pounds. Intermittent fasting has been good for my body and diabetes. Sugar levels are perfect. I am no longer taking any medicine for my diabetes, just intermittent fasting."

- Karen Francka

"Lori has inspired me, encouraged me, and made me think about my routine! Each time in my life that I've had to lose weight, I was a strict calorie counter. I no longer do that...thanks to what I've learned from reading Lori's book! I've also always believed that at my age, it was impossible to lose weight without extreme exercise, but I've lost 14 pounds without stepping outside. So many things have changed for me since I began talking with Lori and fasting. I am no longer a stress eater. I no longer eat just because it's *time to eat*. I no longer crave sweets and junk food. Lori's book has helped me more than you can imagine!!"

- Carol Brakebill

DEDICATION

To my amazing husband, David, and our four awesome kids,
for all their love and support.

DISCLAIMER

I wrote this book based on my personal experience and research with intermittent fasting.

This book is not intended as a substitute for the medical advice of physicians. The reader should consult a physician in matters relating to their health, particularly regarding any symptoms that may require diagnosis or medical attention.

Every effort has been made to ensure the accuracy of the information shared in this book. However, there may be errors. And so, this book should serve only as a general guide, not as the ultimate source on the subject matter.

The author assumes no responsibility or liability for the purchaser or reader of this book.

CONTENTS

COPYRIGHT   2

READER RESULTS   3

DEDICATION   5

DISCLAIMER   7

CONTENTS   9

Introduction   19

Is Intermittent Fasting for You?   23

The State of America's Health   24

How Can Intermittent Fasting Help?   25

This Book Is For You   25

Who This Book Is Not For   26

Is Intermittent Fasting Just a Diet Fad?   28

What Makes This Book Different?   30

Let's Get Started With Intermittent Fasting!   31

How Intermittent Fasting Reversed My Hypoglycemia   35

Reactive Hypoglycemia And A Wake-Up Call   36

How Intermittent Fasting Cured My Hypoglycemia   37

So, What Is Intermittent Fasting Anyway?   39

What Is Intermittent Fasting?   40

Scientifically Proven Health Benefits Of Intermittent Fasting   42

Scientifically Proven Health Benefits of Intermittent Fasting   43

   1. Cellular Repair   43

   2. Weight Loss And Belly Fat Loss   44

   3. Hormone Regulation   44

   4. Lowered Risk Of Type 2 Diabetes   44

   5. Increased Longevity   44

   6. May Help Prevent Alzheimer's   45

   7. Reduced Oxidative Stress And Inflammation   45

   8. Reduced Cholesterol Levels   45

   9. Cancer Prevention   45

Why Intermittent Fasting Is The Simple Way To Lose Weight   48

My Weight Loss Yo-Yo   48

Intermittent Fasting, Losing Weight The Easy Way   52

The Sciency Stuff   52

Simplify Your Life   53

The 5 Most Popular Intermittent Fasting Methods + Schedules   55

Popular Intermittent Fasting Methods   57

   1. The 5:2 Diet - Alternate-Day Fasting   57

   2. OMAD   58

   3. 16/8 Fast (LeanGains)   58

   4. 20-Hour Fast (The Warrior Diet)   59

   5. Meal Skipping   59

Real-Life Examples Of Intermittent Fasting Schedules   60

14/10 Plan - fast for 14 hours / eat within a 10-hour window   60

16/8 Plan - fast for 16 hours / eat within an 8-hour window   61

18/6 Plan - fast for 18 hours / eat within a 6-hour window   61

OMAD Plan - One Meal A Day   61

5/2 Diet Plan   61

Alternate-Day Fasting (ADF) Plan   62

Random Meal Skipping Plan   62

Who Should NOT Do Intermittent Fasting?   64

People Who Should Not Do Intermittent Fasting   64

Women Who Are Nursing Or Pregnant   65

Thin People With Neurodegenerative Conditions   65

People Who Have Eating Disorders   65

Babies And Children   65

Talk To Your Healthcare Provider   66

25 Key Questions About Intermittent Fasting Answered   68

Intermittent Fasting Q&A   68

Q: What is intermittent fasting?   68

Q: What are the benefits of intermittent fasting?   69

Q: Who should NOT do intermittent fasting?   69

Q: How do I start intermittent fasting?   70

Q: What can I eat while intermittent fasting?   70

Q: What can I drink while intermittent fasting?   70

Q: Does intermittent fasting work for weight loss?   71

Q: What are some of the challenges with intermittent fasting?		71

Q: What are some common mistakes people make when intermittent fasting?		71

Q: How do I know if intermittent fasting is working for me?		72

Q: What are some common concerns people have about intermittent fasting?		72

Q: What are some tips for making intermittent fasting easier?		73

Q: What if I'm not losing weight while intermittent fasting?		73

Q: What if I'm not hungry when it's time to eat?		74

Q: What if I'm ravenous while fasting?		74

Q: What should I do if I feel lightheaded or dizzy while fasting?		74

Q: Can I work out while fasting?		75

Q: Won't fasting make me grumpy?		75

Q: I'm worried about losing muscle while fasting. Will I?		75

Q: If I'm fasting in the morning, can I still have my coffee or tea?		76

Q: How challenging is fasting really??		77

Q: How much weight will I lose?		77

Q: Do I have to do IF every day?		78

Q: What's the difference between a diet and intermittent fasting?		79

Q: Will I have trouble concentrating and feel super tired while fasting?		80

**15 Insider Tips For Intermittent Fasting		82**

Tips for Intermittent Fasting Like a Rockstar		82

Stay hydrated by drinking plenty of water.		83

Drink tea and coffee during the fast.   83

Start your fast after dinner.   83

Break your fast with healthy food.   84

Be aware of portion sizes.   85

Listen to your body and eat when you're hungry.   85

Chew your food slowly and savor the flavors.   85

Build up slowly to longer fasts.   85

Don't forget to exercise.   86

Include plenty of protein in each meal.   86

Try IF for at least a month.   86

Be flexible and expect ups and downs.   87

Allow plenty of time for quality sleep.   87

Listen to your body.   87

Be mindful of your eating habits.   88

Top 10 Myths About Fasting, Debunked   90

10 Myths About Intermittent Fasting, Debunked   90

Myth 1: Intermittent fasting is unhealthy.   90

Myth 2: Intermittent fasting is too hard.   91

Myth 3: Intermittent fasting will slow metabolism.   91

Myth 4: Intermittent fasting causes muscle loss.   92

Myth 5: Skipping breakfast is bad for you and will make you gain weight.   92

Myth 6: You must eat small meals to keep your blood sugar under control.   93

Myth 7: Fasting increases cortisol levels.   93

Myth 8: Eating more often speeds up your metabolism.   94

Myth 9: Fasting puts you in "starvation mode," and your body starts
shutting down.   94

Myth 10: You must eat more often to avoid getting hungry.   95

What Is OMAD, And Is It Right For You?   97

What Is OMAD Fasting?   98

OMAD Health Benefits   98

OMAD Fasting Schedule Examples   99

OMAD Precautions And Safety   100

OMAD Research Findings   101

Is it safe to do OMAD every day?   102

Clean Fasting Vs. Dirty Fasting   105

What is clean fasting?   106

Shatter Your Goals With Clean Fasting Foods   107

What is dirty fasting?   107

Avoid These Dirty Fasting Foods   108

My Clean Fasting Vs. Dirty Fasting Experiment   109

The Clean Fasting Experiment Results and What I Learned   110

Symptom Relief and Fasting Benefits   110

A Guide to Fasting and Fitness at Any Age   113

Benefits of Exercising While Fasting   114

Myths About Fasting and Exercise   115

Myth 1: You can't work out while fasting.   116

Myth 2: You need to eat before a workout to have energy.   116

Myth 3: Fasting will make you lose muscle mass.   116

Intermittent Fasting and Exercise: A Perfect Pair   117

What kind of workout should I do when I'm fasting?   118

Exercises You May Enjoy   119

How to Make the Most of Your Workout While Fasting   120

1. Drink plenty of water.   120

2. Warm up properly.   120

3. Don't overdo it.   120

4. Eat a nutritious meal afterward.   120

Insider's Guide To Fasting and Food   123

The Benefits of Eating Healing Foods   124

A Healthy Mindset About Food   125

Intermittent Fasting Nutrition: What To Eat for Maximum Results and
Improved Health   125

1. Bone Broth   125

2. Fermented Foods   126

3. Leafy Greens   126

4. Healthy Fats   126

5. Lean Protein   126

6. Herbs and Spices   126

Healthy Meal Plan Ideas   127

Does Coffee Break a Fast?   131

Coffee Lovers Unite!   132

Black Coffee and Autophagy   132

Does black coffee break ketosis?   133

Benefits of Drinking Black Coffee During Intermittent Fasting   133

Common Questions about Intermittent Fasting and Drinking Coffee   133

Can I have cream and sugar in my coffee while fasting?   134

Does half and half in coffee break a fast?   134

Does almond milk break a fast?   134

Does coconut oil break a fast?   134

Does MCT oil break a fast?   135

Does coffee with milk break a fast?   135

What is the best coffee for intermittent fasting?   135

Will bulletproof coffee break my fast?   135

Can I drink flavored coffee?   136

Other Fasting Friendly Drinks   136

Water   136

Sparkling Water   136

Tea   136

Unsweetened Herbal Tea   137

How To Stay Motivated While Intermittent Fasting   139

Tip #1. Set realistic goals.   139

Tip #2. Find a fasting buddy.   140

Tip #3. Join an online community.   140

Tip #4. Keep a journal.   140

Tip #5. Focus on positive benefits.   141

Tip #6. Visualize better health.   141

Tip #7. Take it one day at a time.   141

Tip #5. Find an inspiring quote.   141

42 Intermittent Fasting Quotes To Inspire You   142

THANK YOU!   146

Appendix A: Bibliography   149

Final Thoughts From Lori   150

Appendix B: Resources   153

About the Author   159

Connect With Lori   161

Introduction

Thank you for purchasing How To Get Awesome Results With Intermittent Fasting: Burn Fat, Lose Weight, and Be Healthy. This version is an update to the original version I wrote in 2017. Since then, I've learned more about intermittent fasting (IF), adding new chapters, including intermittent fasting schedule examples and a meal plan to help you get better fasting results. I love sharing this natural practice and how it has helped me find freedom and improved my health.

At the recent Fasting For Freedom summit hosted by my friend Susannah Juteau, I talked about how intermittent fasting has improved my life in many ways. I shared how it has relieved symptoms caused by chronic disease and helped me to lose weight. I also talked about how it has helped me save time and money and given me more energy to do the things I love.

If you are new to fasting or have been struggling to find a way to make it work for you, I hope this book will be a helpful resource. My goal is to provide you with practical tips, tricks, and examples so that you can experience the many benefits of fasting.

Throughout this book, you'll learn about the tremendous role fasting has played in my journey back to health after a long, debilitating illness. Although I'm not 100% yet, fasting has helped me rise above a complex chronic disease, stronger and more determined than before. I cannot wait to share the excellent health benefits of intermittent fasting with you so you can improve your life too!

This book is an informative yet easy-to-read guide for anyone who wants to learn about intermittent fasting. Whether you are a beginner or you've been fasting for a while, this book is essential for setting the groundwork to help you succeed. The book reveals what IF is and how to use it to your advantage. It also gives you the proven health benefits of IF and debunks common myths. Finally, it answers many questions about fasting and teaches you how to fast like a rockstar, all in a short and easy-to-understand book. Because who's got time to read a novel on fasting?

While researching different eating plans to improve my health, I first learned about IF. I've lived with chronic illness for several years after contracting Lyme disease and tularemia, which went untreated for two years. The illness caused many debilitating symptoms, so I was often bedridden and in pain. Ultimately, I had to quit my teaching job due to the disease.

Extreme fatigue and difficulty focusing on simple activities have been other symptoms of the illness. At times, my short-term memory also suffered. Intermittent fasting has helped me with these issues and much more! It amazes me how much my focus has improved during periods of fasting. My mind is sharper, and my thoughts and memory are clearer. IF even reversed my severe reactive hypoglycemia! As you'll see in the coming chapters, people who practice IF experience these proven benefits. And you can experience all of this for yourself!

I'm grateful to have learned about IF along this health and wellness journey and am excited to share it with you! I only wish I'd found it years ago. Intermittent fasting has helped me lose over 25 pounds with minimal effort after years of weight fluctuations with my pregnancies, breastfeeding, and yo-yo dieting. But more importantly, I no longer deal with the constant cravings for sweets, hunger pangs, and preoccupation with when or what I will eat next.

Fasting has given me tremendous freedom! Freedom from counting calories and being attached to the scale. Freedom to eat what I want to. Freedom from thinking about food all day. Freedom from chronic pain. Freedom from believing that the only way I could lose weight was to eat less and exercise more.

If you are struggling with your weight or health and feel like you've tried everything, intermittent fasting may be the answer you're looking for. Fasting has helped me in many ways, and I know it can help you too! So don't give up hope! The solution may be as simple as eating within a shorter time frame.

Thank you again for buying the book. I cannot wait for you to read this intermittent fasting book and enjoy the excellent health benefits such a natural practice can give you!

Now let's dive in and learn how to use intermittent fasting to improve your health, lose weight, and transform your life!

To your health,

Lori

Is Intermittent Fasting for You?

Kathy is a middle-aged woman struggling with her weight for years. Despite trying every diet and exercise program under the sun, she could never seem to lose more than a few pounds. Plus, Kathy recently learned that she has type 2 diabetes. Her doctor tells her that if she doesn't get her diabetes under control, she could be facing serious health problems down the road.

Kathy feels pretty desperate when she comes across an article about intermittent fasting. She decides to give it a try and starts with a few 16-hour fasts each week. To her amazement, after about three months of intermittent fasting, Kathy has lost 30 pounds! Plus, her blood sugar levels are now well within the normal range.

Kathy is thrilled with her results and is convinced that intermittent fasting is a true miracle. She's now sharing her story with others in the hopes that they will feel inspired to try this fantastic natural practice.

A few months later, Kathy can stop taking her diabetes medication altogether. As a result, she feels healthier and happier than she has in years and can finally enjoy her life to the fullest.

Now, Kathy is passionate about intermittent fasting and determined to help others experience the same excellent results she did. She is convinced that intermittent fasting is the key to unlocking optimal health and wellness for everyone. Thanks to Kathy's personal story, more and more people are now interested in trying intermittent fasting. Who knows? Maybe you will be next!

If you are struggling with your weight or health, I urge you to keep an open mind as you read this book and consider trying intermittent fasting for yourself. I believe that it has the potential to change your life, just as it did mine.

The State of America's Health

Did you know that 41.9% of Americans are obese? The economic cost of obesity is $173 billion per year, based on a 2019 CDC report.

American adults and children struggle more with obesity and associated health problems than ever before. In 2020, the CDC found that 19.7% of children aged 2 to 19 were obese. In addition, type 2 diabetes affects children in the United States earlier than ever.

The American Psychiatric Association (APA) recognizes weight stigma as a mental health disorder. In addition, the APA reports that people who are obese often suffer from low self-esteem, poor body image, and depression.

Obesity is linked to several severe health conditions, including heart disease, stroke, and type 2 diabetes. In addition, people who are obese have an increased risk of developing these conditions.

The statistics are staggering, and they only continue to climb. But there is hope. Intermittent fasting is a powerful tool that can help you lose weight, heal your body, and transform your life.

How Can Intermittent Fasting Help?

Intermittent fasting is a natural approach that offers many health benefits and can simplify your life. However, the results of fasting happen over time. The benefits of fasting will occur when you learn how to start fasting and regularly incorporate the practice into your daily life.

Intermittent fasting is not a quick fix. It's a lifestyle change. It can be challenging to start if you don't have the right tools, but the benefits are worth it.

By embracing intermittent fasting, you can shed those extra pounds and embark on a journey to revitalize your body and reclaim control of your life. It is a natural approach that offers many health benefits and can simplify your life. The results of fasting happen over time. The benefits of fasting will occur when you learn how to start fasting and regularly incorporate the practice into your daily life.

This Book Is For You

This book is for people looking for a natural way to lose weight, heal their bodies, and transform their lives. Intermittent fasting is an approach that offers many health benefits and can simplify your life.

This book is also for people who have struggled with their health, weight, and wellness despite exercising, Western medicine, and following diets and meal plans. Intermittent fasting is a natural approach that can offer many benefits and help people achieve their health goals.

This book may be for you if you want to improve your health and well-being. Intermittent fasting is a safe and effective way to lose weight, heal your body, and transform your life.

Who This Book Is Not For

This book is not for people looking for a quick fix or wanting to lose weight fast. While intermittent fasting can help you lose weight quickly, this book aims to help you develop a sustainable practice that will improve your health and wellness over time.

This book is also not for people unwilling to commit to learning about and incorporating intermittent fasting into their lives. Anything worth doing takes time and effort, including developing a healthy lifestyle. So if you're not ready to commit to making some changes in your life, this book is probably not the right fit for you.

Are you tired of

- Feeling tired?
- Suffering from digestive issues, diabetes, or other chronic illnesses?
- Feeling unwell?

- Carrying around extra weight that you can't seem to lose?
- Do you feel like you've tried every diet, and nothing has worked?

If you answered yes to any of these questions, then intermittent fasting may be the answer you're looking for. Intermittent fasting is not a diet. It's a way of eating with numerous health advantages and can help simplify your life. The benefits of fasting emerge gradually over time. When you learn how to start fasting and integrate it into your daily routine regularly, fasting results will occur.

I struggled with weight and health for years, trying nearly every diet and exercise program. I saw some results, but they were never sustainable or enjoyable. When I finally discovered intermittent fasting, everything changed. I was able to lose weight, heal my reactive hypoglycemia, and improve my overall health (more on that in the next chapter). And best of all, it was simple and sustainable.

Do you want

- More energy?
- Improved digestion?
- Fewer skin problems?
- To lose weight?
- To feel better overall?

I hear you, and I have been there, too. I used to feel tired all the time, despite getting enough sleep. I had digestive issues and was overweight. I tried every diet out there, and while I saw some results, they were never sustainable or enjoyable. When I finally discovered intermittent fasting, everything changed.

Are you ready for

- Better health?
- Fewer cravings?
- A slimmer waistline?
- More energy?
- Less inflammation?
- Less body pain?
- To feel better overall?

If any of this resonates with you, then intermittent fasting may be able to help.

Is Intermittent Fasting Just a Diet Fad?

Some might say that intermittent fasting is nothing more than a diet fad that will not work in the long run. They would also say there is no scientific evidence to support the health claims about intermittent fasting.

However, many studies show the health benefits of intermittent fasting. These benefits include weight loss, improved mental clarity, and reduced inflammation. Intermittent fasting is a safe and effective way to improve your health. It is also a simple practice you can incorporate into your daily life.

I completely understand if you are concerned about IF being just another fad diet. I felt the same way when I first heard about it.

But after doing research and experimenting with IF, I can confidently say that it is not a fad diet but rather a sustainable and healthy eating pattern that offers many benefits for your health and well-being.

One of the reasons why intermittent fasting is so effective is because it helps to reset your body's natural hormone levels. When you eat all the time, your body is constantly in "feast mode" and produces high levels of insulin and other hormones to deal with the constant influx of food. However, when you fast intermittently, your body has a chance to rest and repair itself, and this results in improved hormone balance.

Intermittent fasting also helps to boost your metabolism and promote fat burning. When you fast, your body is forced to use stored energy (fat) for fuel, resulting in weight loss. Additionally, fasting increases human growth hormone levels (HGH), essential for muscle growth and fat loss.

Finally, intermittent fasting has been shown to have numerous other health benefits, including reducing inflammation, lowering blood sugar levels, improving brain function, and reducing the risk of chronic diseases like heart disease and cancer.

If you're ready to try intermittent fasting, I've created this book to help you get started. In the book, I will share with you everything I've learned from years of intermittent fasting, including:

- The basics of intermittent fasting and how to get started
- The science behind why intermittent fasting works
- The different types of intermittent fasting schedules
- How to troubleshoot common issues with fasting

- And much more!

This book is for you if you're ready to start your journey to better health, weight loss, and improved wellness.

I know what it's like to feel trapped in an unhealthy body. I was overweight, felt exhausted all the time, and was struggling with chronic health problems. But I also know what it's like to feel liberated from those problems. When I discovered intermittent fasting, my life changed for the better. And I believe it can do the same for you.

This book is still for you even if you have no interest in weight loss and are perfectly happy with your body. The health benefits of intermittent fasting are vast, and I believe everyone can benefit from this practice.

So, if you're ready to transform your health, body, and life, let's get started!

What Makes This Book Different?

But first, here are four ways this book is different:

- The book includes case studies and personal experiences to help illustrate the benefits of intermittent fasting.
- The book is geared towards beginners, making it easy to understand and follow.
- The book provides helpful tips and tricks for making fasting more accessible and more manageable.
- The book is based on my personal experiences with

fasting. I have used intermittent fasting for years with great success, so I am uniquely positioned to offer this advice.

Intermittent fasting is not a fad diet; it's a sustainable way of eating that can help you lose weight, heal your body, and transform your life. With many health benefits, intermittent fasting may soon become part of your routine. The key to seeing results is consistency with your practice and making it part of your lifestyle.

Intermittent fasting can benefit your health in many ways, including weight loss, reducing inflammation, and improving blood sugar levels. I have seen these benefits in my life, and I believe you can see results, too. With the right approach and a commitment to consistency, intermittent fasting can be a valuable tool in your wellness arsenal.

Intermittent fasting can be a powerful tool to improve your health, but believing in yourself and your wellness journey is essential. Stay consistent with your practice, and make intermittent fasting part of your lifestyle. With time, you'll discover this approach's many benefits and feel proud of your commitment to wellness.

Let's Get Started With Intermittent Fasting!

We all want to live a healthy life, but knowing where to start is hard. Trying to figure out how to eat healthily, exercise regularly, and get enough sleep can be overwhelming. And even if we stick to a healthy lifestyle for a while, it's easy to fall off the wagon when life gets busy.

Intermittent fasting is a simple, effective way to improve your health without feeling like you're depriving yourself or making huge changes to your lifestyle. Instead, you can enjoy eating healthy foods and still indulge in your favorite treats with intermittent fasting.

You can also save money and time because you won't have to prepare special meals or buy expensive supplements. Intermittent fasting is a sustainable, lifelong approach to health that can help you lose weight, heal your body, and transform your life.

Intermittent fasting is a great way to improve your health and simplify your life. By learning how to start fasting and incorporating it into your daily routine, you can reap the many benefits of this practice.

Chapter One Summary:

In this chapter, we addressed who this book is for and who it is not for. If you are looking for a diet book, this is not the book for you. This book is for people who want to live healthier lives and improve their overall health through intermittent fasting.

Intermittent fasting is a simple, effective way to improve your health without feeling like you're depriving yourself or making considerable changes to your lifestyle. Instead, you can enjoy eating healthy foods and still indulge in your favorite treats with intermittent fasting. You can also save money and time because you won't have to prepare special meals or buy expensive supplements.

Intermittent fasting is a sustainable, lifelong approach to health that can help you lose weight, heal your body, and transform your life. By learning how to start fasting and incorporating it into your daily routine, you can reap the many benefits of this practice. In the next chapter, we will discuss how to start this journey. I'll also share how IF reversed my reactive hypoglycemia symptoms and changed my life for the better.

You can find all of the research mentioned in this book in Appendix B: Resources near the end.

How Intermittent Fasting Reversed My Hypoglycemia

Living a healthy life can be challenging. It's overwhelming to figure out how to eat healthily, exercise regularly, and get enough sleep. And even if we stick to a healthy lifestyle for a while, it's easy to fall off the wagon when life gets busy.

Intermittent fasting is a simple, effective way to improve your health without feeling like you're depriving yourself or making considerable changes to your lifestyle. Instead, you can enjoy eating healthy foods and still indulge in your favorite treats with intermittent fasting.

You can also save money and time because you won't have to prepare special meals or buy expensive supplements. Intermittent fasting is a sustainable, lifelong approach to health that can help you lose weight, heal your body, and transform your life.

A few years ago, I began having frequent blood sugar issues. I would eat a meal or snack, then less than two hours later, break out in a cold sweat, feeling weak, dizzy, nauseous, and like I was going to pass out. Maybe you can relate? Many times I was on the verge of fainting with my head between my knees or lying on the couch while my husband offered me a banana with peanut butter to get my sugars back up. So I could function and get back to life. These episodes started coming more often and more intensely. And, with all the other health problems I encountered with untreated Lyme disease, I knew I should get it checked out.

Reactive Hypoglycemia And A Wake-Up Call

My doctor ordered me to take a fasting 3-hour glucose tolerance test. If you've ever been through this, you know the experience takes half a day. First, you have to drink a cold, syrupy (and disgusting) liquid, then wait at the doctor's office, having your blood drawn multiple times at 1-hour intervals to check your glucose levels. I remember feeling okay after the first blood draw and sleepy and sick after the second.

Then, after the third blood draw, I was ready to leave and go home because I felt weak and nauseous. The office was only a 10-minute drive from my house, so I didn't think much of it. But as they say, hindsight is 20/20.

I got in my car and drove about a half mile from the doctor's office when I went around a sharp curve I'd driven many times before, feeling myself fade in and out of consciousness, nearly passing out, driving off the road and almost into a ditch.

It was scary. If I'd known how out of it I truly was, I would never have attempted to drive myself home. But instead, I was thankful I made it home safely and didn't cause an accident. Although it certainly wasn't the best decision I've ever made, it was *a wake-up call.*

As expected, my doctor called a few days later and said my test showed I had reactive hypoglycemia. She asked me how I'd felt after the last blood draw, and I confessed my near-accident. Then she mentioned she didn't know how I drove home because my glucose levels were so low. She introduced me to a special diet for people with hypoglycemia, and I started following it immediately. She also suggested looking into intermittent fasting.

How Intermittent Fasting Cured My Hypoglycemia

I researched natural cures for hypoglycemia and found information about intermittent fasting and how it reduces insulin resistance and can even prevent type 2 diabetes. So, after talking to my doctor, I started the 16/8 IF method and noticed drastic improvements in my health within a few short weeks.

The cold sweats, weakness, constant hunger, and cravings for sweets and carbs dissipated and have continued to improve over time. Fasting has now completely cured my hypoglycemia. I used to have horrible brain fog due to the neurological impact of Lyme. However, IF has helped with that too. Also, I tend to get easily distracted, but during my fasting periods, I'm more focused and better able to concentrate than before. I wish I'd known about IF years ago because it has helped me health-wise in countless ways and simplified my life.

Since I've been practicing IF for several years, I've worked with many people who have used fasting to lose weight and improve their health. So if you're discouraged by health issues or have been a yo-yo dieter for years as I was, keep reading. I've seen many people upgrade their health and life with intermittent fasting, and I'm confident it can do the same for you too!

Chapter Two Summary:

Intermittent fasting is a proven method to help you improve many health problems, including blood sugar issues caused by hypoglycemia. IF has made a fantastic improvement in how I feel and live daily. Whether you want to lose weight, gain muscle or simplify your life, intermittent fasting can help.

If you're unsure of what intermittent fasting is, don't worry! We'll be exploring the concept more thoroughly in the next chapter.

You can find all of the research mentioned in this book in Appendix B: Resources near the end.

So, What Is Intermittent Fasting Anyway?

Alice was always tired. She would wake up feeling achy and drained, no matter how much she slept. She had tried every diet out there, but nothing seemed to work. Her friend kept telling her that she should try intermittent fasting, but she was hesitant.

She finally decided to give it a try and found that it was a lot easier than she thought. She started fasting for 12 hours daily and gradually worked up to 16 hours. After a few weeks, she noticed she had more energy and wasn't as achy. She also lost weight without even trying!

Alice is now a big believer in intermittent fasting and recommends it to everyone she knows. As a result, she feels better than she has in years and can finally enjoy life to the fullest.

If you're tired and run down, intermittent fasting may be just what you need to feel your best. In this chapter, we'll define intermittent fasting and explore how it can simplify your life.

What Is Intermittent Fasting?

Intermittent fasting is an eating pattern. It is not a diet. It's not about *what* you choose to eat. But it's all about *when* you eat (or don't eat). Simply stated, it's eating, or not eating, in a strategic way.

Though it has recently gained an impressive following, it has been around for ages. We were once hunters and gatherers who went for days without food. As a result, our bodies are well-oiled machines designed to withstand feast or famine.

Our modern-day eating habits often center around fast-paced lives. Eating frequent meals and snacks of highly processed and fast foods is the norm for many of us. But this doesn't give your body time to rejuvenate and repair the damage these chemicals can do over time.

So, in many ways, IF is a more *natural* way of eating. And this may appeal to many of you striving for better health.

Best of all, fasting is **simple to do**. And almost anyone can do it. Whether you work in a corporate office, are a full-time parent, commute from home, or are young, middle-aged, or elderly. Again, nearly anyone can do IF.

It's especially popular with some weightlifters and elite athletes because it allows you to maintain muscle while losing fat.

Chapter Three Summary:

Intermittent fasting is a concept that has been around for ages. It is not about *what* foods you choose to eat. But it is all about the *timing* of when you eat and don't eat, cycling between periods of feasting and fasting. And now that you know what it is, let's look at some of the incredible benefits intermittent fasting can give you. Fasting isn't easy, but it **is** simple.

In the next chapter, we'll discover what science says about fasting. Let's get into it!

You can find all of the research mentioned in this book in Appendix B: Resources near the end.

Scientifically Proven Health Benefits Of Intermittent Fasting

In the last chapter, we defined intermittent fasting and explained how it's a natural practice that can simplify your life. Now let's look at some of the research behind it.

Fasting has been around for ages. Many people love fasting because of its health benefits. And some love the way it makes them feel.

Say you were a caveman living in the paleolithic era. Your body would go through cycles of feast and famine out of necessity. You may find it surprising that your body is designed to live this way.

In our modern society, we are bombarded with food 24/7. There's always something to eat, whether it's fast food, junk food, or processed food. Unfortunately, this constant availability of food has led to more people being overweight, obese, and chronically ill than ever before.

Perhaps you've heard you should eat frequent, small meals to keep your metabolism stoked. Unfortunately, in reality, this advice keeps you in 'feast mode' and makes you hungrier (much hungrier) than intermittent fasting.

When you live in constant feast mode, eating frequent meals and snacks as many people do, your body doesn't benefit from the natural repair and rejuvenation it's designed for. I lived this way for years until I learned the truth.

Yes, it may sound counterintuitive, but I urge you to try it yourself and see what you think. I'm convinced you'll experience the fantastic benefits of IF too.

Intermittent fasting not only helps you feel full longer. It has many more health benefits supported by scientific evidence.

I'm a Missouri girl, born and raised. Our state nickname is the "Show Me State" because we are known for our skepticism and need proof before we believe something. If you can relate to this sentiment and need a little more convincing, this next section is especially for you.

Scientifically Proven Health Benefits of Intermittent Fasting

1. Cellular Repair

Although your body works to cleanse and detox, when your diet is poor or you're eating around the clock, it doesn't run like it's supposed to. Living this way wears out your cells, especially the mitochondria, which are recycled during **autophagy**. It's a fantastic process by which the body cleans and repairs old, damaged cells. Fasting gives the body time to focus entirely on necessary repairs. Also, recent research shows the benefits of fasting for Alzheimer's patients.

Next up is one reason so many people turn to fasting.

2. Weight Loss And Belly Fat Loss

IF can boost your metabolism and help you lose weight and belly fat. Losing weight with intermittent fasting causes *less* muscle loss than straight-up calorie restriction.

3. Hormone Regulation

Fasting causes an increase in human growth hormone levels. Consequently, this facilitates fat-burning and muscle gains.

4. Lowered Risk Of Type 2 Diabetes

Intermittent fasting can lower blood sugar levels and decrease insulin resistance. Over 34 million Americans have diabetes, and most cases are Type 2.

Fasting has been shown to reverse type 2 diabetes. As I mentioned in chapter 1, it reversed my severe reactive hypoglycemia, a precursor to type 2 diabetes. This next benefit impacts everyone.

5. Increased Longevity

Studies in rats have shown intermittent fasting extends the lifespan. And though we need human studies to learn more about the impact on humans, these findings are promising.

6. May Help Prevent Alzheimer's

Alzheimer's disease is the most common neurodegenerative disease. Currently, there is no cure. Yet, animal studies show that intermittent fasting may offer protection against neurodegenerative diseases, including Alzheimer's, Parkinson's, and Huntington's.

7. Reduced Oxidative Stress And Inflammation

Studies show that intermittent fasting can protect the body against the harmful effects of oxidative stress and inflammation. This benefit is significant because inflammation in the body increases the risk of many chronic diseases, including heart disease, cancer, Crohn's, and rheumatoid arthritis.

8. Reduced Cholesterol Levels

IF decreases triglycerides and LDL cholesterol. We're talking about bad cholesterol. (Remember, the L in LDL stands for *low* because you want this number to be as low as possible.)

9. Cancer Prevention

Cancer is a horrible disease characterized by the uncontrolled growth of cells. Several studies have shown that IF may help prevent cancer. Evidence also suggests that fasting may cut the side effects of chemotherapy.

Chapter Four Summary:

Recent studies about intermittent fasting have discovered

excellent results. IF can help you lose weight and belly fat, lower cholesterol, reduce oxidative stress and increase human growth hormone. In addition, practicing IF lowers your risk of type 2 diabetes, increases longevity, and may even help prevent cancer and neurodegenerative diseases. These proven health benefits must be making you so excited right about now! I know I'm excited for you and the future you can have with fasting.

As we'll see, intermittent fasting is a simple and natural way to lose weight.

You can find all of the research mentioned in this book in Appendix B: Resources near the end.

Why Intermittent Fasting Is The *Simple* Way To Lose Weight

I realize that using the words **fasting** and **simple** weight loss in the same sentence may seem contradictory. But please allow me to explain with a personal story.

My Weight Loss Yo-Yo

First, I'll share some background about myself. Today I'm focused on growing healthier and stronger. But as a teenager, and like many other young, impressionable girls, I was keenly aware, observing the world around me. And what I learned had an impact on my body image. Though I heard *pretty is as pretty does*, and *beauty comes from the inside*, I also observed people preoccupied with appearances, constantly talking about 'bad' and 'good' foods and focusing on physical attractiveness.

This, combined with societal pressures that girls (and boys) act and look a certain way, creates confusion in young minds. As a result, my relationship with food was not always healthy. I

restricted calories and food groups for years because I believed it was the best thing for me, my weight, and my appearance. But now, thankfully, I enjoy eating until I'm satisfied, and my relationship with food has improved drastically. Not only that, but **thanks to fasting, I'm at a healthy weight, enjoy eating all my favorite foods, and don't have the cravings and hunger pangs I used to.**

In the past, I tried many weight loss programs. As a mama to four beautiful and now grown babies, my body has morphed from thin and frail from Lyme disease to round and nine months pregnant, and everywhere in between (not in that order) more times than I can count. Maybe you can relate in some way?

With each pregnancy, I was extremely nauseated, throwing up, and unable to keep food down for the first several months. As a result, I always lost weight and did not gain in the first half of my pregnancies.

And each time, this would alarm my doctor, so he would tell me to eat more and start putting on weight. At the time, this sounded like an impossible task until nausea let up towards the latter half of the pregnancy. I pressed on full speed ahead then and followed my doctor's orders to a tee.

You can probably see where this is going. With Drew, our first child, I gained 43 pounds in 4 months. For someone who's only 5'6," I thought that must have set some record. However, after he was born, I was so busy breastfeeding on demand and caring for a newborn that I was able to lose all the weight before we found out we were expecting our second-born son, Cooper, 15 months later.

And on it went. The weight went up and down with each little bundle of joy. And as our family grew, at times, so did my waistline. And may I say, our children have been the most amazing blessings, and I wouldn't change a thing (except for the weight loss yo-yo).

So, thank you for indulging in my trip down memory lane. All to say this, *I understand the frustrations and difficulties of wanting to lose weight and putting it off because you think:*

- I'm too busy with my job.
- It's too hard.
- I've tried so many times. Why should this time be any different?
- My family needs me. I'll do it when the kids are older.
- There aren't enough hours in the day.
- I don't want to spend money on a gym membership.
- Fill in the blank with an excuse, ahem, reason.

If you're like me, we can come up with a million excuses about what we want, can't we? And as you can see, I truly understand. *The struggle is real! But,* If I could go back in time, I would approach my weight loss efforts with intermittent fasting.

Why? Because for me, intermittent fasting:

- Makes losing weight so much easier because it's a natural appetite suppressant
- Makes life simpler because less shopping and meal prepping is involved

- Doesn't require you to record what you eat or count points or macros
- Allows you to eat the foods you want and not have to cut out entire food groups
- Boosts my concentration
- Reduces my inflammation and body pain (symptoms of Chronic Lyme disease)
- Improves my short-term memory (another sign of Lyme)
- Eliminates the hunger pangs and cravings I used to get multiple times a day

Since discovering IF, I **no longer live a life of food restriction**. I have the freedom to eat what I want to. I now know that there are no bad or good foods. But I'm in touch with how I feel after I eat certain foods. Knowing that eating whole natural foods makes me feel better and more energized causes me to want to eat more nourishing foods in the future.

On the flip side, if I eat processed food that makes me feel lousy, I don't want to eat as much (or any) of that food anymore. The beauty of fasting is that I have the freedom to choose what foods I eat. IF allows me the freedom to indulge when I choose. Suppose I attend a wedding and I have the opportunity to enjoy a slice of delicious wedding cake with my favorite buttercream frosting. In that case, you'd better believe I will enjoy it.

Because of IF, I can now delay eating the special foods I love when I want them. Or when it's a special occasion or holiday. In the past, I would have denied myself. Or ate the food but felt guilty later.

Intermittent Fasting, Losing Weight The Easy Way

When fasting, your body has to use its stored fat for energy. Using body fat for fuel is good and much more effective than just cutting calories. If you want to lose excess fat, IF is a great way to do it.

So forget what you've heard about eating 3 or 5 or 6 meals a day and keep reading because the calories in, calories out theory does not work.

The Sciency Stuff

I'm not a doctor and don't pretend to be one. However, I've included some excellent books in Appendix A at the back of this book to check out and learn more about the science behind how fasting works. In particular, I'd recommend reading The Obesity Code by Dr. Jason Fung. That said, here is some background on how fasting works.

When you're fasting, your body releases two essential fat-burning hormones:

- Human growth hormone (HGH)
- Norepinephrine (noradrenaline)

HGH can help with fat loss and muscle gains.

When norepinephrine is released, it breaks down body fat into fatty acids, which are burned for energy.

Also, during fasting periods, **insulin** *decreases significantly.* This action leads to fat burning. Fat burning! And more fat burning!

Insulin is the key here. *Eating more raises insulin and causes your body to hold onto fat.*

Conversely, fasting lowers insulin which causes your body to burn fat.

Now put down the beaker, take off your white coat, and exit the lab because we're going somewhere new.

If you've ever thought of living in a tiny house (and even if you haven't), you'll love this next part.

Simplify Your Life

When you eat less often, you have fewer meals to plan. As a result, you have less grocery shopping to do. Not to mention, you spend less money on groceries because you're often eating less food.

Yes, you do need to make healthful choices. But, because you're making healthy choices when you eat, there's **no need** for calorie counting or point tracking. And attending meetings with weigh-ins and complicated point systems is not necessary either. Can you spell F-R-E-E-D-O-M?!

And that hour-long aerobic workout you've been doing every day for as long as you can remember? Feel free to cut back to 2 or 3 days a week for 30 minutes. You might even replace some aerobics with weight training or a workout with kettlebells. So stay active, but keep it fun!

Please notice that I'm not saying counting points or working out every day is wrong or that you shouldn't do it. For example, I still keep a food diary some days because it makes me conscious of what I'm putting into my body. Whatever works best for you is what you should do.

I want to share my success with IF and encourage you to try it yourself. Look at this as a chance to try something new. Something simple that gives you freedom.

Chapter Five Summary:

Intermittent fasting is more accessible than other weight loss plans because you have fewer meals to prepare. Also, there's no need to count calories or keep track of points. Plus, long workouts aren't necessary because, with IF, your body works like a finely tuned machine, and weight loss tends to become more accessible for most people. Your body is working smarter instead of harder.

Let's get down to business now that you know what intermittent fasting is and some of the advantages. The next chapter will introduce you to various types of fasting and flexible schedules so that you can easily add the practice into your life starting as early as today!

The 5 Most Popular Intermittent Fasting Methods + Schedules

Jack has always been a pretty healthy guy. He played sports in high school and college, and even after he graduated, he stayed active by going to the gym and taking long walks with his dog. But as he got closer to his 50th birthday, Jack started noticing that he was gaining weight, and no matter how much he exercised, it was hard to lose.

One day, Jack stumbled upon an article about intermittent fasting. It talked about how fasting could help people lose weight and feel better overall. Intrigued, Jack decided to do some more research on the topic. He read about the different types of intermittent fasting and decided that 16/8 sounded like the best option for him.

At first, it was tough to adjust to not eating for 16 hours straight. But after a few weeks, Jack started to feel better than ever. He had more energy, lost weight effortlessly, and his thinking was clearer than ever. Plus, he didn't have to deprive himself of foods he loved; he just had to be careful about when he ate them. Now that

Jack has been fasting intermittently for a while, he can't imagine returning to his old ways. He's happy with his new body and the benefits that come with it. If you're thinking about trying intermittent fasting, Jack would tell you to go for it! Who knows, you might just feel as amazing as he does.

This chapter will overview some of the most popular intermittent fasting methods. You can use this information to decide which way is best for you, or, better yet, explore them all!

As I shared earlier, IF tremendously benefits your health. Not only can it help you lose weight and belly fat, but it also helps with:

- Cellular repair through autophagy
- Hormone regulation
- Lowering your type 2 diabetes risk
- Preventing Alzheimer's
- Cancer prevention
- Reducing cholesterol
- Reducing oxidative stress and inflammation
- Increased longevity

There are several different ways to do IF. And this is great because everyone is unique, so we don't need a "one size fits all approach." But, if you're like me, you want a plan that fits your personality, style, and life. So in this chapter, I'll teach you some of the most popular intermittent fasting methods. Always keep in mind that you can design IF to fit **your** schedule. Fasting can adjust any way you want it to. This lifestyle is about what works for YOU. That's the beauty of fasting. You make it fit your life and become a lifestyle you will never want to part with.

I will also share several real-life examples of intermittent fasting schedules.

Popular Intermittent Fasting Methods

Here are a few of the most popular intermittent fasting methods.

1. The 5:2 Diet - Alternate-Day Fasting

Alternate-day fasting (ADF), in the truest sense, is where you fast every other day.

Then, on the off days, you eat as you usually would. Some people call the up-day, down-day eating plan.

Another form of ADF is where you only eat 500 calories on fasting days. Then you eat as you usually would on the non-fasting days.

The 5:2 Diet was developed by a British journalist and doctor, Michael Mosley. It's another form of ADF because it involves eating normally five days a week and limiting caloric intake the other two days. During the fasting days, they recommend that women restrict their calories to 500 per day and men to 600 per day.

So, for example, you might choose Tuesday and Thursday as your fasting days. You could enjoy two small meals of 250 to 300 calories each of those days. Or you could eat all your calories in one meal. Then the other five days, you would eat normally.

I tried the 5:2, but it's not for me. I found it too difficult to sustain long-term, and it was hard for me to sleep going to bed feeling hungry. I know some people like it, though, so you might find it a good fit for you too. The best way to learn is by trying it for yourself.

2. OMAD

The One Meal A Day fasting plan is trendy and has some well-known followers, but is it practical or sustainable? OMAD is intermittent fasting that has you eat one meal per day. This could be any meal, at any time during the day, making it a very flexible plan.

Some people choose to do OMAD to lose weight quickly, but this may not be the healthiest way to go about it. If you want to try strict OMAD, it's essential to ensure you get all the nutrients your body needs from that one meal. This can be tough, which is why some people prefer other intermittent fasting methods.

That said, one of the biggest (and favorite!) influencers in intermittent fasting, Gin Stephens says that she does OMAD. However, her approach seems more relaxed and often includes a snack, a meal, and dessert. This approach allows you to get all the nutrients your body needs without feeling deprived. Because you're eating more than a single meal, it's safer and easier to stick to long-term.

3. 16/8 Fast (LeanGains)

The 16/8 is my go-to and was my favorite IF method for years when I first started because it's easy and fits my schedule. And most importantly, it keeps me motivated. Plus, I don't feel like eating when I wake up, so the 16/8 allows me to grab my black coffee and go.

With this method, you fast each day for 16 hours and eat within an 8-hour window. 16/8 is also known as the LeanGains method, which fitness guru Martin Berkhan started.

One way to do 16/8 (popular with many IF-ers) is not to eat after dinner, then skip breakfast the following day. So, for example, if you finish dinner at 7 pm and don't eat your next meal until 1 pm the following day, you've fasted for 16 hours.

4. 20-Hour Fast (The Warrior Diet)

Ori Hofmekler developed the Warrior Diet. The plan here is to fast for 20 hours, then eat one large meal in the evening.

However, something that makes this plan unique is that during the 20-hour fast, you're allowed to eat small snacks of Paleo-friendly foods, such as raw fruits and vegetables, juice, and protein.

I join many fasting purists who say that because of this, The Warrior Diet isn't true fasting at all. However, many people have succeeded, so I'll mention it here.

5. Meal Skipping

You'll want to try different IF methods to find the one that's right for you. For example, meal skipping is a less structured way to fast that some people enjoy. If you don't feel hungry for a meal one day, skip breakfast, lunch, or dinner.

And don't worry about what you may have heard about meal skipping. You will not lose muscle or go into starvation mode.

This is all a myth. Our bodies are adept at going without food for long periods, so skipping a meal or two randomly or regularly is beneficial. So if you're not hungry or too busy to stop and eat, just skip a meal and eat later when you're actually hungry. No worries!

Remember, intermittent fasting is not the same as starving. Not at all!

Real-Life Examples Of Intermittent Fasting Schedules

This section aims to give specific examples of different fasting schedules. Please keep in mind that the beauty of fasting is that you can design the plan that fits **your** life. These are only examples. I want you to experiment with different fasting options to find the one/ones that are right for you.

Discovering the perfect fasting schedule for you may take a little time, but you have your whole life ahead of you, and there's no rush to get everything figured out today. So feel free to focus on clean fasting from the beginning. Then, after fasting for a few days/weeks/months, you can try out different schedules to find the best combination for you!

The sample schedules below show time-restricted eating (TRE) patterns. They focus on different IF schedules for eating all your food for the day.

14/10 Plan - fast for 14 hours / eat within a 10-hour window

- Eat all of your meals between 10:00 a.m. - 8:00 p.m.
- Eat all of your meals between 7:00 a.m. - 5:00 p.m.
- Eat all of your meals between 3:00 p.m. - 1 a.m.

16/8 Plan - fast for 16 hours / eat within an 8-hour window

- Eat all of your meals between 12:00 p.m. - 8:00 p.m.
- Eat all of your meals between 7:00 a.m. - 3:00 p.m.
- Eat all of your meals between 3:00 p.m. - 11 p.m.

18/6 Plan - fast for 18 hours / eat within a 6-hour window

- Eat all of your meals between 12:00 p.m. - 6:00 p.m.
- Eat all of your meals between 8:00 a.m. - 2:00 p.m.
- Eat all of your meals between 4:00 p.m. - 10:00 p.m.

OMAD Plan - One Meal A Day

- 7:00 a.m. – 11:00 a.m.: Open your eating window with a healthy smoothie, and finish eating your main meal by 11:00 a.m.

- 3:00 p.m. – 8:00 p.m.: Open your window with a small snack, followed by your main meal at 5:30 p.m., then finish eating dessert by 8:00 p.m. (This more flexible approach to OMAD is my favorite)

- 5:00 p.m. – 6:00 p.m.: Eat your main meal between 5:00 and 6:00 p.m. (This example is too restrictive to follow long-term.)

- 1:00 p.m. – 4:00 p.m.: Eat your main meal at 1:00 p.m. and finish eating dessert by 4:00 p.m.

5/2 Diet Plan

Eat normally five days a week and "fast" 2 days a week (not technically fasting because you're still eating food on your "fasting" days, but I include it here because it does offer health benefits, it just tends to be more challenging to follow for many people)

- Sunday, Tuesday, Wednesday, Friday, and Saturday - eat normally; Monday and Thursday - Women: 500 calories; Men: 600 calories
- Sunday, Monday, Wednesday, Thursday, and Saturday - eat normally; Tuesday and Friday - Women: 500 calories; Men: 600 calories
- Monday, Tuesday, Thursday, Friday, and Saturday - eat normally; Sunday and Wednesday - Women: 500 calories; Men: 600 calories

Alternate-Day Fasting (ADF) Plan

Up-day (feasting), down-day (fasting); Make sure you always follow a down-day with an up-day.

- Monday, Wednesday, and Friday - up-day (eat normally); Tuesday, Thursday, and Saturday - down-day (fasting all day)
- Sunday, Monday, Tuesday, Thursday, and Saturday - up-day (eat normally); Wednesday and Friday - down-day (fasting all day)
- Sunday, Monday, Tuesday, Thursday, Friday, and Saturday - up-day (eat normally); Wednesday - down-day (fasting all day)

Random Meal Skipping Plan

- Eat breakfast, lunch, and dinner every day except skip breakfast on Monday, Wednesday, and Friday.
- Eat breakfast, lunch, and dinner every day except skip

breakfast and lunch on Tuesday and Thursday.

- Eat breakfast, lunch, and dinner every day except skip dinner on Monday, Tuesday, Thursday, and Friday.

Chapter Six Summary:

Fasting can simplify your life because you spend less time prepping meals and shopping for groceries. In this chapter, we've covered 5 of the most popular intermittent fasting methods. Remember, there is no right or wrong way to do IF. You might want to try a couple of different methods before you find the one (or ones) you like the best. The beauty of fasting is that you can design it to fit your life and schedule.

If you're just starting, you may want to start with something less demanding, like the 14/10 or 16/8, before trying an OMAD fast. Later in the book, there will be more on adjusting your body to fasting schedules gradually.

Now that you have some practical tools and a better understanding of how intermittent fasting works, you may wonder if the practice could work for you. For example, can everyone intermittently fast, or are there certain types of people for whom it's not recommended?

The good news is that intermittent fasting is generally safe for most people. However, there are a few exceptions, which is precisely what we'll explore next.

Ready to jump in? Let's go!

You can find all of the research mentioned in this book in Appendix B: Resources near the end.

Who Should NOT Do Intermittent Fasting?

In the last chapter, we saw many examples of popular fasting schedules. Now that we know a bit more about how fasting works and the different types of fasting, let's explore who should avoid the practice.

As much as intermittent fasting can benefit some people, it is not suitable for everyone. Therefore, certain people should avoid intermittent fasting or speak to a healthcare professional before trying it.

Fasting is a stressor on the body, and while the practice can be very beneficial for some, it can be detrimental for others. Therefore, avoiding intermittent fasting or speaking with a healthcare professional is best if you have the following conditions.

People Who Should Not Do Intermittent Fasting

According to Dr. Eric Berg, the following groups of people should NOT attempt intermittent fasting.

Women Who Are Nursing Or Pregnant

Babies need ongoing nourishment for the proper growth and development of their brains, organs, and bodies. Based on research, IF can be harmful to babies still in the womb and should therefore be avoided. Depriving yourself or your baby of essential nutrients could negatively impact your child's growth, and it's simply not worth the risk. So, don't do intermittent fasting when you're pregnant.

Thin People With Neurodegenerative Conditions

Dr. Berg explains that this group of people would benefit from a ketogenic diet that is very low in carbohydrates while eating three meals per day. This includes thin people with Alzheimer's, MS, and other neuro conditions.

People Who Have Eating Disorders

Intermittent fasting is inappropriate for people dealing with anorexia, bulimia, or other eating disorders.

Babies And Children

Babies need to be fed on demand. This means they must be fed whenever they are hungry to ensure proper growth and development. IF is not recommended for small children because they demand more nutrition than adults.

Talk To Your Healthcare Provider

Although there are a few exceptions, it's always best to check with your physician before trying a fast, primarily if you identify with any of the above categories.

For instance, when I was diagnosed with reactive hypoglycemia, I was surprised when my doctor suggested I try intermittent fasting. I thought fasting might exacerbate my condition, but she explained that the opposite was true.

If you have any doubts, please don't hesitate to speak with your healthcare professional before trying intermittent fasting.

It has been a few years since I started fasting nearly every day for health reasons. I don't know what I did before I found intermittent fasting! I've tried other diets and health regimens, but fasting is the key to feeling my best.

Please be aware that I didn't proceed with this transition hastily. (I will explain how I did it later in the book.) However, fasting stabilizes my blood sugar, and it's now within a normal range. In addition, IF has successfully reversed my reactive hypoglycemia!

Chapter Seven Summary:
In this chapter, we explored who should avoid the practice of intermittent fasting. Intermittent fasting is not suitable for everyone. Women who are nursing or pregnant, thin people with neurodegenerative conditions, people with eating disorders, babies, and small children should not try intermittent fasting. If you have a chronic health condition, please talk to

your doctor to see if intermittent fasting is right for you.

In the next chapter, I'll answer several common questions about intermittent fasting to help you increase your understanding of this practice. Let's get started!

You can find all of the research mentioned in this book in Appendix B: Resources near the end.

25 Key Questions About Intermittent Fasting Answered

Intermittent fasting is a hot topic in the health world right now. But like any diet or health trend, there are a lot of misconceptions and unanswered questions about it.

This chapter will explore 25 critical questions about intermittent fasting to help you understand it better. After reading this chapter, you'll learn more about intermittent fasting, whether it's right for you, and how to answer any questions.

So let's dive in and answer some of the most pressing questions about intermittent fasting!

Intermittent Fasting Q&A

Q: What is intermittent fasting?

A: Intermittent fasting is an eating pattern that cycles between periods of fasting and eating. It doesn't specify which foods you should eat but when you should eat them. There are many different types of intermittent fasting, but the most popular is 16/8 intermittent fasting. A 16/8 involves fasting for 16 hours and eating during an 8-hour window.

Q: What are the benefits of intermittent fasting?

A: There are many potential benefits of intermittent fasting, including:

- Weight loss
- Improved mental clarity
- Reduced inflammation
- Cellular repair
- Belly fat loss
- Hormone regulation
- Reduced risk of type 2 diabetes
- Reduced oxidative stress
- May protect against neurodegenerative diseases, including Alzheimer's, Parkinson's, and Huntington's
- Increased longevity
- Reduced triglycerides and LDL cholesterol, the "bad" cholesterol
- Possible cancer prevention

Please visit the Appendix B Resources section at the back of this book to access all of today's cutting-edge studies on intermittent fasting, cited in the text.

Q: Who should NOT do intermittent fasting?

A: Women who are pregnant or nursing, thin people with neurodegenerative conditions, people with eating disorders, babies, and small children should not try intermittent fasting. If you have a chronic health condition, please talk to your doctor before trying intermittent fasting.

Q: How do I start intermittent fasting?

A: It's best to start slowly with intermittent fasting and increase your fasting window gradually. For example, if you're used to eating three meals a day, you can start by eating breakfast later and later, eventually pushing it back to 10 or 11 am. Then you can begin fasting from dinner one night until breakfast the next day.

After this, you may want to try skipping breakfast a few days a week and fasting for 24 hours once or twice a month. Once you're comfortable with this, you can increase the frequency and duration of your fasts.

Q: What can I eat while intermittent fasting?

A: There are no strict rules about what to eat while intermittent fasting. However, eating healthy, whole foods during your eating window is generally recommended. This means eating plenty of vegetables, fruits, lean proteins, and healthy fats.

Q: What can I drink while intermittent fasting?

A: Non-caloric beverages are generally allowed while fasting, including water, black coffee, and tea. You can also drink calorie-free seltzer waters and other sparkling waters. However, please avoid sugary drinks, alcohol, and juices while fasting.

Q: Does intermittent fasting work for weight loss?

A: Yes, intermittent fasting can help with weight loss. One of the main reasons some people try intermittent fasting is for weight loss. When you fast, your body burns stored sugar (glycogen) for energy, which leads to weight loss.

In my opinion, weight loss is nice, but the real value of intermittent fasting comes from all of its other benefits.

Q: What are some of the challenges with intermittent fasting?

A: There are a few challenges that people may face when starting intermittent fasting, such as hunger, irritability, and low energy. However, these side effects typically go away after fasting for a few days or weeks.

Q: What are some common mistakes people make when intermittent fasting?

A: Some common mistakes include not drinking enough water,

not getting enough sleep, and overeating during the eating window.

Q: How do I know if intermittent fasting is working for me?

A: There are a few ways to measure whether intermittent fasting is working for you.

First, you can track your weight loss if that is one of your goals. Second, you can track your overall feelings, energy levels, and mental clarity. Third, you can measure health markers, such as blood sugar, cholesterol, and inflammation levels.

Q: What are some common concerns people have about intermittent fasting?

A: Some common concerns include feeling hungry and low on energy. However, these side effects typically go away after fasting for a few days or weeks.

Others are concerned about nutritional deficiencies. If you're eating nutrient-rich whole foods during your designated eating window, you likely don't need to worry about missing out on critical nutrients unless you're fasting for days.

Finally, some people are concerned about the impact of intermittent fasting on their social life. I understand this concern, but there are ways to manage it. For example, you can fast when you know you won't be around food, such as when you're sleeping or at work. Or, you can schedule your fasting days around social events so that you're not missing out.

Q: What are some tips for making intermittent fasting easier?

A: Here are a few tips that may make intermittent fasting easier:

1. Drink plenty of water and unsweetened tea or coffee. This will help you stay hydrated and help reduce hunger.
2. Get enough sleep. Sleep is crucial for overall health and can help reduce hunger levels.
3. Eat nutrient-rich whole foods during your eating window. This will help you feel satisfied and help reduce cravings.
4. Schedule your fasting days around social events. This will help you stick to your fasting plan and avoid feeling left out.
5. Have a plan for breaking your fast. This will help you avoid overeating and help you stick to your goals.

Q: What if I'm not losing weight while intermittent fasting?

A: If you're not losing weight, you can do a few things.

First, ensure you drink plenty of water and unsweetened tea or coffee in your fasting window.
Staying hydrated will help you feel full and may help reduce hunger.

Second, try eating more nutrient-rich whole foods during your eating window. This will help you feel satisfied and help reduce cravings.

Third, make sure you're getting enough sleep. Sleep is crucial for overall health and can help reduce hunger levels.

Finally, consider speaking with a healthcare professional to rule out any underlying health conditions affecting your weight.

Q: What if I'm not hungry when it's time to eat?

A: It's normal to feel a little bit hungry when you first start intermittent fasting. However, as your body adjusts, you should begin to feel less and less hungry. If you're still not hungry after a few days, you can try breaking your fast a little earlier or eating more during your eating window.

Q: What if I'm ravenous while fasting?

A: If you're ever feeling famished while fasting, it's probably best to break your fast early. Intermittent fasting is not about starving yourself – it's about finding the best balance for you.

It's essential to listen to your body's hunger cues and eat when you're truly hungry. Getting in tune with what your body needs will help you avoid overeating and make it easier to stick to your fasting schedule in the long run.

Q: What should I do if I feel lightheaded or dizzy while fasting?

A: If you ever feel lightheaded or dizzy while fasting, please drink some water and eat a small snack. This usually takes care of the problem quickly. However, if you continue to feel dizzy or lightheaded, it's best to break your fast and have a full meal.

Q: Can I work out while fasting?

A: Yes, you can – and many people find their workouts more effective when fast. However, it's essential to listen to your body and not push yourself too hard. If you're feeling weak or tired, it's best to take a break or have a small snack.

Try going for a walk or doing some gentle stretching while fasting. Then, as you get more experience with fasting, you can experiment with different workouts to see what works best for you.

Q: Won't fasting make me grumpy?

A: It's normal to feel a little bit cranky when you first start fasting. However, as your body adjusts, you will likely begin to feel more energetic and clear-headed. If you're still grumpy after a few days, you can try breaking your fast a little earlier or eating more during your eating window.

Q: I'm worried about losing muscle while fasting. Will I?

A: It's unlikely you will lose muscle while intermittent fasting – as long as you eat enough protein, healthy fats, and vegetables during your eating window. Fasting may actually help you build muscle by increasing your growth hormone levels and improving your body's ability to use fat for fuel.

If you're worried about losing muscle, you can always experiment with shorter fasts at first. Then, once you get used to intermittent fasting, you can increase the length of your fasts. In addition, try lifting weights or doing bodyweight exercises while fasting to help you maintain muscle mass.

Q: If I'm fasting in the morning, can I still have my coffee or tea?

A: The short answer is yes! You're free to have water, black coffee, and unsweetened tea. Also, don't miss Chapter 11 about Clean and Dirty Fasting, where we give you a full rundown of what you can have while fasting.

Black coffee and unsweetened tea are great options because they're calorie-free and won't break your fast. Coffee may even enhance the benefits of fasting by increasing fat burning and improving mental clarity. Just be sure to avoid adding sugar or cream, which would add calories and break your fast.

If you're new to fasting, you might wonder how you'll make it through the day without food. Many people find that once they get used to intermittent fasting, they enjoy the increased energy and focus that comes with it. If you're struggling initially, remember that you can always start with a shorter fasting window and work your way up. And be sure to drink plenty of water and get enough sleep to help your body adjust.

Q: How challenging is fasting really??

A: I love this question - it makes me smile! I hope that didn't sound insensitive because I had the same question when I first started. I can genuinely say that fasting is not easy but simple. Depending on how frequently you're fasting, it might take a few days or weeks to get used to your new routine. After getting used to the new schedule, I realized that IF was a better way to live. The pros of this practice outweigh any negatives I initially felt.

It is normal to feel some hunger pangs and cravings as your body adjusts to the new schedule. As a result, your energy might be a little low at first, and you might get a dull headache for the first couple of days. Or maybe not. And truth be told, any symptoms I had were nothing compared to how I felt before I discovered IF. For me, these symptoms were minimal because I adjusted the timing schedule very slowly each day. I'll show you exactly how I did this later in the book!

Hunger pangs and cravings are normal as your body adjusts to intermittent fasting. Initially, your energy might be low, and you might get a headache during the first few days. But don't worry, any symptoms are nothing compared to how you felt before you discovered IF. For me, these symptoms were minimal because I adjusted the timing schedule *very slowly* each day. I'll show you exactly how I did this later in the book!

Q: How much weight will I lose?

A: This is a great question that I'm sure many people want to know! The amount of weight you lose will depend on many factors, including your starting weight, how strict you are with your fasting schedule, and what type of fasting you're doing.

In general, those who are overweight or obese can expect to lose more weight than those who are already at a healthy weight. And if you're doing intermittent fasting to lose weight, aim to create a calorie deficit by eating fewer calories than you burn.

Some people lose a lot of weight very quickly when they start intermittent fasting, while others lose weight more slowly. How quickly you lose weight will also depend on your starting weight and how strict you are with your fasting schedule.

If you're doing intermittent fasting for other reasons than weight loss, such as improving your health or increasing your energy levels, you may still lose some weight. But don't worry if weight loss isn't your primary goal. Intermittent fasting has many other benefits that are worth pursuing!

Q: Do I have to do IF every day?

A: No, you don't have to do IF every day. You can choose which days of the week you want to fast and how many hours each day.

Some people prefer to do a circadian rhythm fast (12/12) or 16/8 fast every other day, while others find it more sustainable to fast for two or three days in a row, then take a break for a day or two. Ultimately, it's up to you to figure out what works best for your body and lifestyle.

There are no right or wrong answers regarding how often you should do IF. Listen to your body, and be flexible with your fasting schedule. You might find that your needs change over time, and that's okay!

Q: What's the difference between a diet and intermittent fasting?

A: As shown below, Dr. Michael Eades provides a well-crafted answer to this question:

"Diets are easy in the contemplation, difficult in the execution. Intermittent fasting is just the opposite — it's difficult in the contemplation but easy in the execution. Most of us have contemplated going on a diet. When we find a diet that appeals to us, it seems as if it will be a breeze to do. But when we get into the nitty-gritty of it, it becomes tough. For example, I stay on a low–carb diet almost all the time. But if I think about going on a low–fat diet, it looks easy. I think about bagels, whole wheat bread, jelly, mashed potatoes, corn, bananas by the dozen, etc. — all of which sound appealing. But were I to embark on such a low–fat diet, I would soon tire of it and wish I could have meat and eggs. So a diet is easy in contemplation but not so easy in the long-term execution. Intermittent fasting is hard in the contemplation, and of that, there is no doubt. "You go without food for 24 hours?" people would ask incredulously when we explained what we were doing. "I could never do that." But once started, it's a snap. No worries about what and where to eat for one or two out of the three meals per day. It's a great liberation. Your food expenditures plummet. And you're not particularly hungry. Although it's tough to overcome the idea of going without food, once you begin the regimen, nothing could be easier."

- Dr. Michael Eades

Q: Will I have trouble concentrating and feel super tired while fasting?

A: It is common to experience some difficulty concentrating and feel tired while fasting, especially in the beginning. This is normal and usually goes away after a few days or weeks of fasting. If you're having trouble concentrating, try drinking more water and adding some Himalayan pink salt or sea salt to your water to replenish electrolytes (sodium, potassium, magnesium). Also, make sure your getting enough sleep, not doing high-intensity workouts (during your fast), and taking breaks throughout the day

Most people notice an energy and mental acuity increase after their bodies have adjusted to fasting. This is also my experience. Remember, though, that you may experience a slow shift towards these benefits at the start of your fasting journey.

Chapter Eight Summary:
In this chapter, we answered some of the most common questions about intermittent fasting, including how to get started, what to expect, and how to make fasting work for you.

We've also dispelled some myths about fasting and shown you that it is a safe and effective way to improve your health. I hope this Q&A chapter has helped answer your questions about IF.

In the next chapter, we'll discuss some practical tips and tricks to help you make the most of your intermittent fasting journey.

There's no time like the present to start feeling your best!

You can find all of the research mentioned in this book in Appendix B: Resources near the end.

15 Insider Tips For Intermittent Fasting

In the previous chapter, we answered some of the most common questions about intermittent fasting. In this chapter, we'll explore some insider tips to help make your intermittent fasting journey as successful as possible.

These tips will help you to:

- Choose the right intermittent fasting protocol for your goals
- Maximize the benefits of intermittent fasting
- Minimize any potential adverse effects

Follow these tips, and you'll be well on your way to achieving outstanding results with intermittent fasting.

Tips for Intermittent Fasting Like a Rockstar

Try these ideas if you're starting intermittent fasting or need a refocus. They aren't hard and fast rules but insider secrets that will push your momentum from the start.

Stay hydrated by drinking plenty of water.

Intermittent fasting can be a great way to boost your energy, lose weight, and feel better. But, first, it's essential to stay hydrated and drink plenty of water. Doing so will help keep hunger pangs away and ensure you get the necessary electrolytes. For example, try drinking 16 ounces of fresh water first thing in the morning and continue throughout the day. You may also want to add a pinch of pure sea salt or Himalayan pink salt to your water for an extra electrolyte boost.

Drinking plenty of water is essential for good health, whether fasting or not. Drink 8-10 glasses of water daily, and even more if you're exercising. You might also want to try herbal tea or sparkling water with a squeeze of lemon for a refreshing change. Just be sure to avoid sugary drinks like juices, sodas, and alcohol.

Drink tea and coffee during the fast.

Caffeine can help suppress hunger pangs and increase energy levels. So, enjoy unsweetened tea and black coffee during your fast. Just be sure to avoid adding milk or sugar, as these can break the fast.

Green tea is an excellent option as it contains polyphenols that decrease hunger and increase satiety. Matcha, in particular, is a concentrated green tea with even more polyphenols. So, if you're looking for an energy boost, try sipping on some matcha during your fast.

Start your fast after dinner.

After dinner is the easiest time for many people to begin their fast because you'll be sleeping most of the time. So there's no reason to make it hard on yourself, right?

One of the best ways to ease into intermittent fasting is to start fasting after dinner. This means you would finish your last meal of the day and not eat again until late morning the next morning. So, for example, you could have dinner at 6 pm and then not eat breakfast until 10 or 11 am the next day.

If this isn't possible, figure out what will work with your schedule. The beauty of fasting is that you decide what works best for you.

Break your fast with healthy food.

Make sure your day's first meal includes plenty of nourishing whole foods. Eliminate processed junk food and sugar as much as possible.

After an overnight fast, your body will welcome nutrients from healthful foods.

Good options for breaking your fast include:

- A smoothie made with nutrient-rich ingredients like fruits, vegetables, and protein powder
- Oatmeal with fruit and nuts
- A healthy omelet or frittata
- A salad with roasted chicken or fish
- Vegetable soup and a sandwich

Enjoying high-fiber, nutrient-rich foods when you break your fast will help you maintain energy levels and avoid overeating later in the day.

If you get hungry before your next scheduled meal, reach for a healthy snack like nuts, seeds, fruit, or raw vegetables. Avoid processed foods and snacks like candy, cookies, or chips as much as possible.

Be aware of portion sizes.

Fasting is not an excuse to overeat when you do eat. Instead, be mindful of portion sizes, especially if you're trying to lose weight. A general rule of thumb is to fill your plate with half vegetables, a quarter protein, and a quarter healthy carbohydrates like fruit, whole grains, or starchy vegetables.

Listen to your body and eat when you're hungry.

One of the best things about intermittent fasting is that it teaches you to listen to your body's hunger cues. If you're feeling ravenous, it's probably time to eat. On the other hand, if you're not hungry, there's no need to force yourself to eat.

Another benefit of intermittent fasting is that it can help you become more aware of when you're hungry and just eating out of habit. Learning to differentiate between the two can help you make healthier choices overall.

Chew your food slowly and savor the flavors.

Don't eat more than you would in a typical meal. Just because you're fasting doesn't mean you can go overboard. On the contrary, overeating will make you feel sluggish and could lead to weight gain. Instead, take time to chew your food slowly and savor the flavors. This will help you feel fuller faster.

Build up slowly to longer fasts.

If you're new to intermittent fasting, start with shorter fasts, like 12 or 14 hours. Once your body gets used to this, you can gradually begin to fast for 16 hours or more.

And if you're really up for a challenge, you could try a 24-hour fast once or twice a week. Just be sure to listen to your body and eat when hungry.

Don't forget to exercise.

Just because you're fasting doesn't mean you have to sit on the couch all day. Exercise is a great way to boost energy levels, improve mood, and promote weight loss.

Just because you're fasting doesn't mean you have to sit on the couch all day. Exercise is a great way to boost energy levels, improve mood, and promote weight loss.

Try to get at least 150-300 minutes of moderate exercise each week. If that's not possible, start with 10-15 minutes a day and build up. And if you don't have time for a full workout, even a 10-minute walk can make a difference.

Include plenty of protein in each meal.

Protein is a great appetite suppressant and essential for maintaining and building muscle. So when you're fasting, include plenty of protein in each meal. Good protein sources include lean meats, fish, tofu, legumes, eggs, and dairy.

Also, include healthy fats like avocados, nuts, and seeds. Healthy fats will help you feel fuller longer and promote better blood sugar.

Try IF for at least a month.

Practicing intermittent fasting for a few weeks gives your body the chance to get used to the new schedule. Additionally, it gives you time to assess the benefits and determine how you want to proceed. If this is something you're interested in exploring further, I'll go into more depth later about gradually easing yourself into a new routine.

Be flexible and expect ups and downs.

It's natural to go through ups and downs in life. Focus on relaxing through these moments, and remember that everything will pass. If possible, get some fresh air and do something you enjoy. Keep learning about IF and focusing on the beautiful changes you're making for your health.

The more you know about intermittent fasting, the more likely you will succeed in your efforts. This means there will be days when you feel great and others when you feel less than stellar. But as long as you continue practicing IF, these bad days will become fewer and far between.

Allow plenty of time for quality sleep.

Intermittent fasting can lead to feelings of fatigue, especially in the beginning. This is normal and will usually pass after a few days or weeks. In the meantime, make sure you're getting plenty of quality sleep.

To get deep, restful sleep, follow these tips:

- Avoid caffeine and alcohol during the hours before bed.
- Create a relaxing bedtime routine.
- Turn off electronics at least 30 minutes before sleep.
- Make sure your bedroom is dark, quiet, and cool.
- Take a hot bath or shower before bed.

Each person is different, but most adults need between 7 or more hours of quality sleep per night.

Listen to your body.

Pay attention to your energy levels, moods and emotions, hunger and food cravings, and overall feelings. Fasting is the perfect time to get in touch with your body's cues.

Take a break from fasting if you're feeling exhausted, irritable, or hungry. There's no need to push yourself harder than necessary. Just return to fasting when you're feeling ready.

Be mindful of your eating habits.

Intermittent fasting is an opportunity to be more mindful of your eating habits. When you eat, pay attention to your food and savor each bite.

This doesn't mean you must spend hours cooking or eating gourmet meals. Instead, be present while you're eating and enjoy the experience of nourishing your body.

You might even find that intermittent fasting improves your relationship with food. For example, when you're no longer eating out of habit or because you're bored, you can start to appreciate food more.

Chapter Nine Summary:

Intermittent fasting is a powerful tool, but it's not a miracle cure.

Just like with anything else in life, intermittent fasting won't work if you don't put in the effort. So, to see the desired results, it would be ideal if you were consistent and dedicated. But we all know that ideal isn't always possible.

The good news is that even if you're not perfect, you can still reap many benefits of intermittent fasting. Just remember to be patient and give yourself some grace along the way.

So there you have it! These are some of my top tips for starting with intermittent fasting. I hope this has been helpful and that you'll give IF a try. Remember, even if you're not perfect, you can still reap many benefits from this practice. Just be patient and give yourself some grace along the way.

I hope these fasting tips help you when you decide to go for it and begin your journey! Different approaches work for various people, but many people experience improved concentration, fantastic weight loss results, fewer sugar cravings, and many more health benefits. So follow these tips to gain the most from your IF experience, and you'll be a fasting expert soon!

In the next chapter, we'll examine the top myths about intermittent fasting. You'll learn the truth about some of the most common misconceptions about this practice. Stay tuned!

You can find all of the research mentioned in this book in Appendix B: Resources near the end.

Top 10 Myths About Fasting, Debunked

In the last chapter, we covered some of the top tips for starting with intermittent fasting. But before you begin your IF journey, it's important to dispel some of the myths that might be holding you back.

This chapter will debunk some of the most common misconceptions about intermittent fasting. After reading this, you'll better understand how this practice can benefit your health and well-being. Let's get started!

10 Myths About Intermittent Fasting, Debunked

These are some top myths about intermittent fasting and why they're false.

Myth 1: Intermittent fasting is unhealthy.

One of the most common misconceptions about intermittent fasting is that it's unhealthy. People often think not eating for extended periods will lead to nutrient deficiencies or other health problems. But the truth is that intermittent fasting is safe for most people and beneficial for your health.

There are many evidence-based health benefits of intermittent fasting. For example, research shows that fasting boosts weight loss, improves insulin sensitivity, and reduces inflammation. Additionally, it can help increase lifespan and protect against chronic diseases like heart disease, cancer, and Alzheimer's disease. So if you're worried that intermittent fasting is unhealthy, don't be! This practice can help improve your overall health and well-being.

You'll find all of the research mentioned in this book under Appendix B near the back of the book.

Myth 2: Intermittent fasting is too hard.

Another common myth about intermittent fasting is that it's too difficult to stick with. People often think they can't go without food for long periods or that they'll be too hungry. But the truth is that intermittent fasting is not as hard as it seems. Intermittent fasting becomes much easier with time. After a few days or weeks of fasting, your body will adjust, and you won't feel as hungry.

Many people find that their hunger decreases during fasting periods. If you're worried about being too hungry while fasting, try starting with a shorter fasting period, like a 12-hour circadian rhythm fast. Once your body adjusts, you can gradually increase the length of your fasting periods. Additionally, drink plenty of water and enjoy black coffee and unsweetened tea during your fasting periods to help reduce hunger.

Myth 3: Intermittent fasting will slow metabolism.

One of the biggest concerns people have about intermittent fasting is that it will slow their metabolism. They think that not eating for extended periods will cause their body to go into "starvation mode" and burn fewer calories. But the truth is that intermittent fasting actually boosts metabolism.

Intermittent fasting helps boost metabolism by increasing human growth hormone (HGH) levels. HGH is a hormone that helps regulate metabolism, muscle growth, and fat loss.
So if you're worried about your metabolism slowing down during intermittent fasting, don't be! On the contrary, this practice may help speed up your metabolism.

Myth 4: Intermittent fasting causes muscle loss.

Some people believe that when we fast, our bodies burn muscle and use it for fuel. Though this is true with dieting in general, there's no evidence showing that this happens specifically with intermittent fasting. Instead, the evidence suggests that IF is superior for maintaining muscle mass. Pretty cool, huh? In one study comparing IF to daily caloric restriction, both resulted in similar weight loss; however, those practicing IF showed much less reduction in muscle mass.

So what does this all mean? It means you can intermittently fast without worrying about losing your hard-earned muscle mass. Phew!

Myth 5: Skipping breakfast is bad for you and will make you gain weight.

Skipping breakfast may not be as bad for you as you think. A 2014 randomized controlled trial compared a group of 283 overweight and obese adults eating breakfast versus those skipping breakfast. After the 16-week study, the two groups had no difference in weight.

So, what does this mean for you? First, intermittent fasting may be a good option if you're trying to lose weight. Skipping breakfast may help you reduce your daily calorie intake and lead to weight loss.

Of course, everyone is different, and you should always listen to your body. For example, it may be best to eat breakfast if you're feeling famished in the morning. But if you're not feeling hungry, skipping breakfast may be an excellent way to help you optimize your health and achieve your weight loss goals.

Myth 6: You must eat small meals to keep your blood sugar under control.

Despite what many diet "experts" say, you don't need to eat small meals throughout the day to support energy and be mentally efficient. And this is because blood sugar is well-regulated in healthy people.

Are you aware that your blood sugar is regulated by ghrelin and other metabolic hormones? And, more often than not, it imitates the eating patterns you're accustomed to.

Believe it or not, people can quickly adapt to periods of fasting. You don't have to eat often to control your blood sugar because it adapts to your regular meal patterns just fine. It's how your body was designed.

Myth 7: Fasting increases cortisol levels.

Cortisol is a steroid hormone that is produced by the adrenal glands. It often gets a bad rap, but it has many vital roles in the human body. For example, cortisol helps control blood sugar, regulates metabolism, works as an anti-inflammatory, and influences memory formation and blood pressure.

One critical study found that short-term or intermittent fasting causes cortisol to drop. So please don't worry about fasting and increasing your cortisone. It simply is not valid.

Myth 8: Eating more often speeds up your metabolism.

Many believe that if they eat more often, their metabolism will speed up, causing them to lose weight. Although your body does burn a small number of calories while digesting food, it's not very significant. This process is scientifically called the thermic effect of food (TEC).

Research has shown that the body expends the same number of calories whether you eat all your calories in 2, 3, 5, or 6 meals daily. The important thing is to keep insulin levels low (through fasting) because this causes fat burning.

Myth 9: Fasting puts you in "starvation mode," and your body starts shutting down.

This myth has been around for years; unfortunately, many people still believe it. But the truth is that intermittent fasting can help speed up your metabolism! Any long-term weight loss will cause the body to burn fewer calories. And when you weigh less, you have fewer calories to burn. That's why, if you've tried losing weight on a point system, such as Weight Watchers, after you've lost some weight, your points decrease.

Studies show fasting for up to 48 hours can boost your metabolism by 3.6 to 14%!

However, your metabolism can slow down if you fast longer, so keep this in mind.

Myth 10: You must eat more often to avoid getting hungry.

Some people say eating snacks helps ease their hunger and avoid cravings. And others find that eating less often keeps them satisfied longer. In this case, it seems they're both right. There have been several studies on this, and they've had mixed results. Some studies suggest eating more frequent meals, and snacks causes increased hunger, others find no effect, and others show an increase in appetite.

I feel more hungry the more I eat, and eating snacks makes me more hungry. Fasting in between meals keeps me feeling satisfied and virtually eliminates thoughts of food and cravings.

Chapter Ten Summary:

As you know, intermittent fasting is a popular and efficient approach to losing weight and improving your health. However, as you can see, there are several misconceptions about fasting. It's beneficial to deconstruct these myths so you can relax while fasting without worrying about the small stuff. As you know, many people have benefited from IF; I am confident you will too! Knowing the facts about fasting will help empower you on your journey.

In the next chapter, we'll look at OMAD, or "one meal a day," a type of intermittent fasting in which you eat all your calories for the day in one meal. Are you up for the challenge? I think you are! Let's do this!

You can find all of the research mentioned in this book in Appendix B: Resources near the end.

What Is OMAD, And Is It Right For You?

Intermittent fasting can be a great way to lose weight and improve your health, but what if you want to take things one step further? What if you're interested in trying one meal a day fasting, also known as OMAD? This type of fasting involves eating all your daily calories in one meal (or close to it). Is this right for you? Let's find out!

OMAD is popular with many intermittent fasters. It stands for *one meal a day*. After several years of doing the 16/8, 18/6, 20/4, and a few 36-hour fasts, I decided to try OMAD and find out for myself. I discovered that OMAD has its place, and I try to do a 24-hour fast (or 2) each week.

I like to mix things up to keep life interesting (so my body doesn't get used to one particular fasting schedule), so most weeks, I do a combination of an OMAD, a couple of 20/4s, 18/6s, and 16/8s to keep my body guessing.

This is the beauty of fasting. It gives you the freedom to choose when you want to fast within the structure of your day. I tend to be more relaxed and go with the flow, and fasting has helped me get back in touch with my body's cues. I don't deny myself nourishing real food. If I feel hungry before my fasting window closes, I'll eat something delicious and healthy.

My husband, David, has been practicing OMAD periodically too. He usually does it a couple of days a week and has noticed several benefits within the short time since he's started, including

- Weight loss
- Improved body composition
- Fewer cravings for sweets
- Increased energy

What Is OMAD Fasting?

OMAD is a form of intermittent fasting. You may have heard it called the One Meal A Day diet. (I don't like using the word *diet* because it implies restriction to me, and I want to focus on what I can have instead of what I can't have.) Simply put, you eat one meal a day and fast for the other hours.

You can have water, unsweetened tea, and black coffee during the fasting window.

OMAD Health Benefits

There are several compelling benefits of including OMAD in your fasting roundup. Many of them are similar to the fasting benefits I shared earlier, but with OMAD, they're magnified. Here are a few.

- People have reported impressive weight loss.
- Autophagy, the recycling of old cells, shifts into overdrive.

- It saves money because you're eating less often.

- You have even less hunger and cravings.

- It saves time because when you're only eating one meal a day, your time spent in the kitchen prepping food for meals is significantly reduced.

- People report increased energy and focus - and who doesn't love being more productive? (When you're OMAD-ing, you don't have to deal with that after-lunch brain fog that happens when your body is busy digesting a meal.)

- Research shows that OMAD time-restricted feeding lowers body mass and fat mass while increasing fatty acid oxidation during exercise without impairing aerobic capacity or strength.

OMAD Fasting Schedule Examples

With OMAD, you have flexibility. Most people doing OMAD eat within a time-restricted eating (TRE) window of 2 to 4 or 5 hours. Here are a few examples of OMAD fasting schedules. Keep in mind that these aren't set in stone. I just created them on the fly to give you some idea of what OMAD can look like:

- 7:00 a.m. – 11:00 a.m.: Open your eating window with a healthy smoothie, and finish eating your main meal by 11:00 a.m.

- 3:00 p.m. – 8:00 p.m.: Open your window with a

nourishing snack, followed by your main meal at 5:30 p.m., then finish eating by 8:00 p.m. (my favorite schedule for OMAD fasting)

- 5:00 p.m. – 6:00 p.m.: Eat your main meal between 5:00 and 6:00 p.m. (not advised more than once or twice a week)
- 1:00 p.m. – 4:00 p.m.: Eat your main meal at 1:00 p.m. and finish eating by 4:00 p.m.

So, if you decide to try OMAD, make it your own. Choose the schedule or schedules your body responds to best, and don't worry about what everyone else is doing, fasting-wise.

It can take a while to figure out which fasting schedule (or schedules) you like the best. So have fun experimenting with different ones and testing how you feel and how your body responds.

OMAD Precautions And Safety

Although OMAD has some great benefits, it's not for everyone and needs to be approached cautiously. I've read a few posts from women who have experienced hormone issues and hair loss they believe was connected to prolonged OMAD, so this is something to be aware of. Please remember that hair loss can happen when you lose a lot of weight (but it generally grows back).

Gin Stephens is a huge proponent of OMAD and says she follows this fasting schedule most of the time. There are many other people who are living the OMAD lifestyle and loving it too.

I like Gin's take on OMAD because it's flexible. She listens to her body's needs (great advice for us all), and if she's feeling hungrier one day, she might add a snack, enjoy dessert, or extend her eating time.

OMAD Research Findings

Although there isn't a tremendous amount of research on the long-term effects of OMAD, I found a couple of things worth sharing. One study found that type 2 diabetes patients saw **improved blood sugar** counts after trying OMAD.

Another study compared two groups of normal-weight people over six months. One group ate one meal a day, and the other ate three. The research found that the people in the one meal a day group lost body fat despite maintaining weight. They also experienced increased blood pressure and total, LDL and HDL cholesterol.

I have seen some excellent OMAD health benefits for myself and my husband when it's used less frequently. (And it sure is nice to have fewer dishes to clean up.) It has helped many people lose weight, lower their insulin levels, and upgrade their overall wellness.

As I mentioned earlier, my experience with OMAD is not a

consistent daily OMAD. I like to switch up my fasting schedule to keep my body guessing. This approach works great for me, but you may prefer something different. So find what works best for you.

Is it safe to do OMAD every day?

It depends on the approach. If you have a single plate of food every day, and that's it, you're going to miss out on essential vitamins and minerals your body needs.

So, if you're underweight or suffer from nutritional deficiencies, you might do better switching up your timing schedules to make sure you're eating enough healthy foods.

Because I have been healing from chronic illness and my doctor says my body doesn't do a great job absorbing nutrients, I like to use OMAD as an occasional approach, but not every day.

Talk to your healthcare provider so they can guide you based on your specific health requirements.

Chapter   Eleven   Summary:

I hope this has given you a good understanding of OMAD. Eating one meal a day is an intermittent fasting schedule you may want to look into, especially if you've been fasting for a while and want to boost your weight loss, simplify your life, or are ready for more of a challenge. Many people have seen great success and experienced additional relief from their symptoms while practicing OMAD. You may find that you love OMAD too.

You can find all of the research mentioned in this book in Appendix B: Resources near the end.

Clean Fasting Vs. Dirty Fasting

Liam had always been interested in fasting. He had read all the books and tried all the different methods. He had even worked up to three 16/8 fasts a week, but it was tough, and he didn't feel that great. But he kept hearing about how great intermittent fasting was and how it could help him lose weight, have more energy, and think more clearly. So he decided to give it another try.

In the past, when Liam woke up, he'd pour himself a cup of coffee and add a little bit of his favorite creamer. He'd heard that this was okay, but he was beginning to doubt whether or not it was helping him. So he decided to just drink water and black coffee in his fasting window for a week and see how he felt.

The first few days were tough. Liam had headaches and felt a little lightheaded, but he pushed through. By day four, he started to feel better. His energy levels were up, and his head was clear. He was even losing weight! He was so excited that he decided to keep going.

A few weeks later, Liam felt terrific. He had lost 15 pounds, his cravings were gone, and he had endless energy. He was even thinking about trying a longer fast. Intermittent fasting completely changed his life, and he was never going back.

If you're like Liam and interested in intermittent fasting, it's essential to understand the difference between clean and dirty fasting. First of all, clean fasting is the only way to go. This means abstaining from all food and drinks that contain calories during your fasting window. That means no coffee with creamer, no juices or sodas, and no snacks.

Clean fasting will help you get the most out of your fast, and you'll see the best results.

I've been experimenting with the benefits of clean and dirty fasting in recent months. I wanted to get some helpful information and share it with you. Below is a rundown of everything I've learned through trial and error. Hopefully, my research will provide beneficial information for your fasting journey!

What is clean fasting?

When I started fasting years ago, I'd never heard of clean or dirty fasting. But to say clean fasting is not essential would be an understatement. Clean fasting creates the ideal fasting environment - one without any insulin spikes.

Some of the key benefits of clean fasting include enhanced fat burning and tremendous overall success. As its name suggests, clean fasting involves consuming only calorie-free, unsweetened (and no artificial sweeteners) drinks.

Shatter Your Goals With Clean Fasting Foods

So, what food items can you eat while clean fasting? The foods listed below are the only ones that have been proven safe. They won't cause your insulin levels to spike and will help promote fat burning, which we all want to achieve.

- Black coffee
- Water
- Unsweetened tea
- Sparkling water
- Herbal teas, not fruit-flavored

What is dirty fasting?

I'm so glad you asked. According to Gin Stephens, dirty fasting does not exist because if you're not fasting clean, then you're not fasting at all. I couldn't agree more! Dirty fasting is when you consume foods or beverages that break your fast. Some experts will tell you dirty fasting is fine. And to be honest, I didn't know there was a difference for years because much of what I read said you were still fasting as long as you keep your calories under 100 during your fasting window.

So, I had my bulletproof coffee every morning and still experienced some of the benefits of fasting, including better mental clarity, improved energy, elimination of my reactive hypoglycemia symptoms, and effortless weight loss of over 25+ pounds. But let me tell you that once I started practicing clean fasting, I experienced a noticeable shift in benefits and additional weight loss.

When I started clean fasting, I realized it was easier to stick to the fast. Because my body didn't have to release insulin every time I drank my creamy coffee or chewed sugar-free gum, I hardly felt hungry, and cravings became a distant memory. So, if you are fasting for weight loss and have hit a plateau (or simply aren't seeing the results you'd like), try clean fasting for better results. I'd love to know what you discover!

Avoid These Dirty Fasting Foods

Technically, any food will break your fast, but the ones listed below are common culprits, otherwise known as "dirty fasting" foods. Eating any of these foods will spike your insulin and stall your weight loss, especially if you're eating or drinking all day, even in very small amounts.

- Coffee creamer
- Cream
- Milk
- Almond milk or any other type of milk
- Artificial and natural sweeteners, including Stevia
- Lemon slices
- Collagen powder
- Protein powder
- Sugar-free sodas
- Sugar-free breath mints

- Sports drinks
- Sugarless gum

Now, let's take a quick look at my clean fasting experiment and see what we can learn from it.

My Clean Fasting Vs. Dirty Fasting Experiment

When I started my clean fasting experiment, I had one goal: to test the effects of clean fasting on weight loss and overall well-being and see if it made a difference for me. After all, I'd been struggling to lose those last 10 pounds for months and felt frustrated.

To begin with, I'd like to clarify one thing for everyone interested: I'm not a scientist and don't pretend to be one on TV. *I'm just a girl who loves fasting and occasionally geeks out over research, facts, and figures that may be useful.* So please take this information with a grain of salt. The only test subject was me. Even though this may be true, the results are still compelling.

My clean and dirty fasting experiment was simple and carried out over a couple of weeks. I focused on the following factors:

- My symptom relief and the benefits of fasting
- My ketone levels (how quickly I got into ketosis with fasting alone, not by a keto eating plan) or fat-burning intensity

The Clean Fasting Experiment Results and What I Learned

Symptom Relief and Fasting Benefits

The benefits I experienced from clean fasting outweighed those of dirty fasting. I felt considerably more focused, had greater energy (which I still battle due to chronic Lyme), and felt little hunger. My brain was sharp, and I was efficient. In addition, my body was benefiting from the higher-level benefits of autophagy, the cell regeneration process.

I used my fasting app to track my fasting time accurately and measured my ketone levels in the afternoon before breaking my fasting using Keto Strips. On the days I did clean fasting, I entered ketosis earlier in the day and was in deep ketosis, as shown by the deep purple color on the Keto Strips. On the other hand, if I entered ketosis on the dirty fasting days, it was always in the trace to small ketone amounts. These results showed me that clean fasting put me in fat-burning mode faster and at a deeper level than dirty fasting.

Chapter Twelve Summary:

I hope this chapter helped you see the difference clean fasting can make in your overall results. These superior fasting results are incredibly apparent if you're trying to lose weight. So if you've been fasting for a while and find your weight loss has stalled, ensure that you're clean fasting to improve your results!

The next chapter will explore how exercise can perfectly complement intermittent fasting. Stay tuned to get all the details!

You can find all of the research mentioned in this book in Appendix B: Resources near the end.

A Guide to Fasting and Fitness at Any Age

Mia was always trying to find the best way to improve her health. She had three young kids and wanted to be able to keep up with them, run around at the park, and feel good in her own skin. She had heard about intermittent fasting and decided to give it a try.

She started by gradually adding more fasting days each week and found that she enjoyed it. Mia also started walking in nature, which she found peaceful and calming. The combination of intermittent fasting and nature walks helped her improve her health and strength while enjoying the process.

The natural practice fit easily into her schedule, and she felt more energized and focused. She also noticed that her clothes fit better and had more energy to play with her kids. Fasting alone gave her more energy and clarity of mind, but adding nature walks to the mix made her feel even better.

Mia's story is just one example of how you can combine intermittent fasting and fitness to optimize your health and well-being at any age.

In the last chapter, we learned about clean fasting and why it's essential for fasting success. Now, we're going to dive deeper into fitness and how it relates to fasting. We'll cover everything from how to start working out again after a long break to how to modify your workouts while fasting. We'll also dispel some common myths about fasting and exercise, such as the idea that you can't work out while fasting or need to eat before a workout to have energy. By the end of this chapter, you'll have a clear understanding of how to approach fitness while intermittent fasting and how to make it work for you at any age.

Whether you're an intermittent fasting pro or fasting for the first time, you may wonder if and how this lifestyle will mesh with your workouts. Or if it's even safe to work out at all in a fasted state.

The great news is that you can continue your fitness regimen. Fortunately, as it turns out, exercising in a fasted state has several health benefits that I'm sure you'll appreciate.

Benefits of Exercising While Fasting

Did you know that working out and fasting can cause oxidative stress on your muscles? It may sound bad, but it's actually beneficial in this case.

Fitness expert Ori Hofmekler explains that acute states of oxidative stress are:

" … essential for keeping your muscle machinery tuned. Technically, acute oxidative stress makes your muscle increasingly resilient to oxidative stress; it stimulates glutathione and SOD [superoxide dismutase, the first antioxidant mobilized by your cells for defense] production in your mitochondria along with increased muscular capacity to utilize energy, generate force, and resist fatigue.

Hence, exercise and fasting help counteract all the main determinants of muscle aging. But there is something else about exercise and fasting. When combined, they trigger a mechanism that recycles and rejuvenates your brain and muscle tissues."

Exercising in a fasted state can help you:

- Burn fat
- Lose weight
- Improve body composition
- Boost cognitive function
- Increase growth hormone

All great reasons to work out before breakfast!

Now, let's address some common myths about exercise and intermittent fasting.

Myths About Fasting and Exercise

Here are some of the most widespread misconceptions about fasting and exercise:

1. You can't work out while fasting.

2. You need to eat before a workout to have energy.
3. Fasting will make you lose muscle mass.

Let's debunk each of these myths one by one.

Myth 1: You can't work out while fasting.

This is simply not true. Many people find that working out while fasting helps them to have more energy and focus during their workouts. When you're used to eating before a workout, your body burns the calories from the food you just ate instead of burning fat. When you fast before a workout, your body is forced to burn fat for energy, leading to more effective workouts.

Myth 2: You need to eat before a workout to have energy.

Eating before a workout can be counterproductive, leading to blood sugar spikes and crashes that leave you tired and unfocused. When you're fasting, your body is in a state of ketosis, which means burning fat for energy, often providing more stable energy levels throughout your workout.

Myth 3: Fasting will make you lose muscle mass.

The myth that fasting will lead to muscle mass loss is disproven by emerging evidence, which shows that fasting has many health benefits beyond just weight loss. In addition, for athletes, there may be potential new ways to maintain performance while in the fasted state.

It's best not to push yourself too hard to exercise in a fasted state, especially when you're first starting. Just as with anything new, it's essential to ease into it and listen to your body. If you feel like you don't have the energy to push yourself hard, take a break or cut your workout short. You can always try again tomorrow.

Remember, there are no rules when it comes to fasting. Everyone is different, so find what works best for you and go with it. Trust your body, and be patient as you experiment to find what works best for you.

Some days, you may feel strong and able to do a hard workout, while others may feel like you need to take it easy. That's perfectly normal and to be expected. But, most importantly, you're listening to your body and doing what feels best for your health and fitness goals.

Intermittent Fasting and Exercise: A Perfect Pair

Intermittent fasting and exercise are a perfect pair because they both help to optimize your health. Fasting helps to improve insulin sensitivity, increase growth hormone levels, and promote cell repair, while exercise helps to improve cardiovascular health, increase muscle mass, and reduce body fat.

When you combine the two, you're giving your body the best of both worlds: the benefits of fasting and the benefits of exercise.

If you're new to intermittent fasting, it's best to approach a fasting workout cautiously. Start with a shorter fasting window, such as 12 hours, and gradually increase the amount of time you fast as you become more comfortable with it.

It's also essential to ensure you're eating enough during your eating windows. Eating too little can lead to fatigue and low energy levels, making it challenging to complete a workout.

Additionally, it's essential to stay hydrated when you're fasting. You'll need even more water to replace the fluids you lose through sweat while working out. Drinking plenty of water throughout the day will help to keep your energy levels up and prevent dehydration.

Finally, remember that, although fasting and exercise are healthy practices, they are also stressors on your body. Be sure to listen to your body and give yourself time to recover between workouts. Taking a day or two off each week will help your body to heal and prevent burnout.

Go for it if you feel better eating something before you work out. But, if you're looking to maximize the benefits of fasting, consider working out in a fasted state and see how your body responds.

What kind of workout should I do when I'm fasting?

One of the best things about working out while intermittent fasting is that you can do any workout you want! Whether you prefer cardio, strength training, or a combination of both, you'll be able to reap the benefits of exercising while fasting.

If you're new to fasting, however, you may want to start with lower-intensity workouts. This will help you get used to the feeling of working out in a fasted state and avoid any potential lightheadedness or dizziness.

As you become more comfortable with fasting, you can increase the intensity of your workout. Just listen to your body, and don't push yourself too hard. Fasted workouts are not the time to PR!

Exercises You May Enjoy

If it's been a while since you've worked out, or if you're new to fitness, here are a few exercises you may enjoy:

- Walking
- Hiking
- Biking
- Swimming
- Yoga
- Pilates
- Light weightlifting
- Bodyweight exercises (squats, lunges, push-ups, etc.)
- Rowing

Remember, the goal is to move your body and get your heart rate up, so choose an activity you enjoy and can sustain for 30 minutes.

How to Make the Most of Your Workout While Fasting

Now that we've answered the question "Can I work out while fasting?" it's time to learn how to make the most of your workout in a fasted state. Here are a few tips to help you get the most out of your training:

1. Drink plenty of water.

This is important any time you work out, but it's especially crucial when fasting. Be sure to drink plenty of water before, during, and after your workout to avoid dehydration.

2. Warm up properly.

A proper warm-up is a key to any good workout. A light 5-10 minute warm-up will help get your blood flowing and prepare your body for exercise.

3. Don't overdo it.

As we mentioned before, fasting is not the time to PR. Listen to your body, and don't push yourself too hard. You may have less energy than usual, so it's essential to take it easy.

4. Eat a nutritious meal afterward.

Once you've completed your workout, consider eating a healthy meal or snack to replenish your energy stores if you feel hungry. This will help you recover from your workout and prepare for your next fast.

These simple tips can help you make the most of your workout while intermittent fasting. Just remember to listen to your body and go at your own pace. With some planning, you can make the most of your fasted workouts and see excellent results.

Chapter Thirteen Summary:

Fasting is a perfectly safe and normal way to approach fitness, whether you're just starting or are a seasoned athlete. If you have questions or concerns about implementing fasting into your fitness routine, speak with an intermittent fasting coach, healthcare provider, or certified fitness professional.

In the next chapter, we'll learn about nourishing foods to eat during your eating windows when you're intermittent fasting. Don't forget to fuel your body to support your fitness goals!

You can find all of the research mentioned in this book in Appendix B: Resources near the end.

Insider's Guide To Fasting and Food

Jenny was always in a hurry. She had a chronic illness that made it difficult for her to move around, so she was always running late. To make matters worse, she loved junk food and ate it all the time because it was fast and easy. Her doctors told her she needed to start eating healthier, but she just didn't think she had the time.

One day, Jenny heard about intermittent fasting and decided to try it. She was amazed at how easy it was to follow and, within a few weeks, started feeling much better. She lost weight, had more energy, and started thinking more clearly. Seeing all the improvements encouraged her to start making time to prep healthy meals so she could continue feeling her best.

If you're like Jenny and are always on the go, intermittent fasting is a great way to improve your health without making big changes to your lifestyle. And although you may not have a lot of extra time, making an effort to fuel your body with nutritious foods in your eating window can make a big difference in how you feel. So, don't be afraid to use fasting as a springboard for more healthy habits. This chapter will show how you can incorporate healing foods into your fasting lifestyle to help support your health goals.

The Benefits of Eating Healing Foods

Most of what you've read has focused on when to eat or not eat. That's because this is what intermittent fasting is all about. Many people will tell you that you can eat whatever you want and still lose weight while intermittent fasting.

This may resonate with some people, but if you want to be as healthy as possible, I recommend eating healthier and making better choices whenever possible. To clarify, I'm not suggesting you deprive yourself of the foods you love. I don't limit my favorite foods that aren't considered healthy, such as fried chicken, coconut cake, or pizza. But, on the other hand, I don't eat them every day. And even if I did, I wouldn't feel so wonderful.

I focus on eating roughly 90% nutritious foods and allowing myself the other 10% for less healthy foods. However, for me, this isn't a hard and fast rule. I'm flexible with it. Some days the ratio of healthy to unhealthy foods may be more like 98%:2%, 70%:30%, or depending on the day, event, and situation, (dare I say) 50%:50%. #RealLife

I'll confess that I generally feel awful after a day of eating less healthy food. Junk food only worsens my symptoms. So, I often do a longer fast the day after I indulge because it's restorative and revitalizing. You may discover this is true for you too.

A Healthy Mindset About Food

It's all a matter of mindset. I adore eating healthy, micronutrient-dense foods that nourish my body because of the way they make me feel. When I eat crummy junk food, I feel crummy. Hence the saying, you are what you eat. Maybe you can relate to this quote also.

We're talking about nourishing your body with real, wholesome food. Plus, healthy nutrition is crucial if you're aiming to lose weight, gain muscle mass, protect yourself from disease, and radiate health and vitality.

So, with that in mind, below are some general tips to guide your food choices and maximize your results while intermittent fasting.

Intermittent Fasting Nutrition: What To Eat for Maximum Results and Improved Health

When you're intermittent fasting (and even if you're not), it's essential to focus on eating whole, unprocessed foods that are rich in nutrients and fiber. These nutrient-dense foods will help fill you up and give you sustained energy throughout the day. Here are some of our favorite healing foods to eat.

1. Bone Broth

Bone broth is rich in minerals and amino acids that support gut health, detoxification, and immunity. It's also a great source of collagen, which benefits skin, hair, and nails.

2. Fermented Foods

Fermented foods are a great way to add healthy probiotics to your diet.

3. Leafy Greens

Leafy greens are packed with vitamins, minerals, and antioxidants. They're also a great source of fiber, which helps promote regularity and healthy digestion.

4. Healthy Fats

Healthy fats are essential to a nutritious diet and help promote satiety. Good sources of healthy fats include avocados, olive oil, nuts, and seeds.

5. Lean Protein

Lean protein is a vital part of a healthy diet and helps support muscle growth and repair. Good lean protein sources include chicken, fish, tofu, and legumes.

6. Herbs and Spices

Herbs and spices are not only delicious but also offer numerous health benefits. They're a great way to flavor your food without adding salt or sugar.

These are just a few healing foods you can incorporate into your diet to support your intermittent fasting lifestyle. Remember, the key is to focus on whole, unprocessed foods rich in nutrients. By doing so, you'll be sure to reap all the benefits of intermittent fasting and improve your overall health.

Healthy Meal Plan Ideas

This is a one-week healthy meal plan option. These dishes and snacks may be modified to fit your fasting routine. Perhaps you're following a specific eating plan, such as Paleo, Keto, Vegan, Whole 30, or gluten-free. Or, you may simply be trying to eat more healthily and cleanly.

For the purpose of this example, I focused exclusively on nutrient-dense meals and snacks because fasting allows for more food freedom (instead of restriction). However, feel free to customize this sample plan to fit your particular nutritional requirements. This is merely an example to inspire you to integrate more wholesome foods into your meals.

Breakfast: Eggs, bacon, ½ an avocado, and berries
Lunch: Greek salad with feta cheese, olives, and cucumbers
Dinner: A simple sheet-pan meal with chicken breast, sweet potato, red pepper, onion, and broccoli tossed in olive oil.
Snack: Pecans and dark chocolate

Breakfast: Green smoothie with spinach, banana, almond butter, berries, and coconut or almond milk

Lunch: Taco cauliflower rice bowls
Dinner: Beef chili with fresh veggies and hummus
Snack: Homemade guacamole with fresh veggies

Breakfast: Spinach omelet with bell peppers and cheese
Lunch: Nitrate-free turkey breast slices on sourdough bread with tomato and avocado with fresh garden salad and oil and vinegar dressing
Dinner: Pork tenderloin, steamed broccoli, and wild rice
Snack: Granny Smith apple, sliced with almond butter

Breakfast: Overnight oats with chia seeds, nuts, and fruit
Lunch: Burrito bowl with black beans, quinoa, and vegetables
Dinner: Grilled salmon, sweet potato, and steamed broccoli
Snack: Homemade peanut butter balls with flax seed

Breakfast: Baked oatmeal with berries
Lunch: Asian chicken lettuce wraps
Dinner: Big salad steak, blue cheese, and tomatoes
Snack: Plain Greek yogurt, frozen cherries, and honey

Breakfast: Protein pancakes topped with almond butter and berries
Lunch: Peanut butter and honey sandwich on sourdough bread
Dinner: Grilled shrimp with greens cooked with bacon and apple cider vinegar
Snack: Homemade granola with nuts and seeds

Breakfast: Avocado toast on sourdough with fresh herbs, Himalayan pink salt, and cracked black pepper
Lunch: Buddha bowls with tahini sauce, sweet potatoes, kale, chickpeas, and brown rice

Dinner: Tacos with ground beef or chicken, cheese, tomatoes, lettuce, salsa, and cilantro
Snack: Red bell pepper with homemade guacamole

Chapter Fourteen Summary:

It is essential to nourish your body with wholesome food, including protein-rich foods, healthy fats, and antioxidant-rich fruits and vegetables. Avoid sugary, simple carbohydrates and prepackaged foods. And perhaps, most importantly, drink plenty of water.

You will succeed more with intermittent fasting if you focus on nourishing your body with nutrient-rich foods. This will help to improve your overall health and well-being. Many healthy meal plan options are available, so find one that fits your lifestyle and dietary needs (or create your own). And be sure to drink plenty of water!

In the following chapter, we'll look at a popular beverage and how it complements the fasting lifestyle. Ready to dive in? Let's go!

You can find all of the research mentioned in this book in Appendix B: Resources near the end.

Does Coffee Break a Fast?

In the last chapter, we looked at nourishing foods, and I shared an example meal plan to give you some ideas. Remember, there are no hard and fast rules when it comes to intermittent fasting – you can adjust and tailor the approach to fit your own needs and preferences.

I often get asked whether coffee breaks a fast, so I wanted to address that in this chapter. I know it's hard to believe that I could write an entire chapter about coffee, but trust me – it's worth it!

Coffee is a popular drink, and everyone has their own opinion about it. For example, some people say that coffee doesn't break a fast, while others believe it does. So, what's the truth?

The short answer is that it all depends on what you put in your coffee. If you add milk or sugar, then yes, coffee will break a fast. However, if you drink black coffee, it technically doesn't break a fast.

Of course, there's a bit more to it than that. So let's take a closer look at the different types of coffee and how they affect fasting. We'll also answer common questions about fasting, drinks, and coffee.

Coffee Lovers Unite!

Coffee is a great way to start the day – it's energizing and can help you to feel more alert. For many of us, it's also a delicious treat! However, if you're fasting, you might wonder if coffee is off-limits.

Coffee consumption is a normal part of many morning routines, and it's often consumed during a fasting window. But does coffee break a fast?

The short answer is no; black coffee will not break your fast. However, if you like to drink black coffee, it can help you reach your desired intermittent fasting goals. Coffee can help you feel more alert and focused, which can be helpful when you're trying to stick to a fasting protocol. Additionally, coffee can help to boost your metabolism and increase fat burning.

Black Coffee and Autophagy

Autophagy is the process by which your body breaks down and recycles damaged cells. It's useful for cellular repair and linked to increased longevity. Fasting is one of the best ways to promote autophagy. Coffee has caffeine which can also help to promote autophagy, making it a great choice to drink during a fasting window.

Does black coffee break ketosis?

Ketosis is a metabolic state in which your body uses fat for fuel rather than carbohydrates. Some people follow a ketogenic diet to reach health goals such as weight loss. Black coffee will not break ketosis. Coffee can help you achieve and maintain a state of ketosis.

Benefits of Drinking Black Coffee During Intermittent Fasting

Black coffee is high in antioxidants, has many health benefits, and is an excellent choice to drink during fasting. Coffee can help you feel more alert and focused, boost metabolism, and promote autophagy. Additionally, black coffee will not break ketosis. So if you're looking for a healthy beverage to drink during your fasting window, black coffee is a great option.

Common Questions about Intermittent Fasting and Drinking Coffee

Now that we know black coffee won't break a fast, let's explore other popular questions about intermittent fasting, coffee, and common add-ins.

Can I have cream and sugar in my coffee while fasting?

Coffee by itself is a great way to start your day during intermittent fasting. However, many people enjoy their coffee with cream or sugar. While black coffee is OK to have while fasting, adding cream and sugar to your coffee can break your fast. This is because a splash of milk and cream contains calories and fat, which will be digested by your body and may kick you out of fasting mode.

Does half and half in coffee break a fast?

Adding half and half to your coffee may make it taste creamy and delicious, but it will also break your fast. So if you'd like to enjoy half and half in your coffee, it's best to drink it after you've broken your fast for the day.

Does almond milk break a fast?

Almond milk is plant-based milk made from almonds. It's a popular choice for coffee but can also break your fast. This is because almond milk contains calories and fat, which your body will digest.

Does coconut oil break a fast?

Coconut oil is a delicious fat that may offer health benefits. Some people believe it can help with weight loss, but no scientific evidence supports this claim. So, does coconut oil break a fast?

The answer is yes. Coconut oil is a source of fat and calories and will therefore break a fast.

Does MCT oil break a fast?

MCT oil is a concentrated source of medium-chain triglycerides (MCTs), a type of saturated fat. MCTs are believed to be a more efficient energy source and may help boost metabolism. So, does MCT oil break a fast? You can probably already guess, but the answer is yes. This is because MCT oil contains calories and fat, which will be digested and may kick you out of fasting mode.

Does coffee with milk break a fast?

I love drinking a delicious mocha latte or cappuccino when I'm not fasting. But if you're fasting, adding dairy milk or plant-based milk to your coffee can break your fast.

What is the best coffee for intermittent fasting?

As you may have guessed, black coffee is the best coffee to drink while intermittent fasting. Black coffee is high in antioxidants and has many health benefits. Additionally, coffee can help you feel more alert and focused, boost metabolism, and promote autophagy.

Will bulletproof coffee break my fast?

Yes, bulletproof coffee will break your fast. Bulletproof coffee is a high-fat coffee drink that includes butter or coconut oil. You can enjoy bulletproof coffee after you've broken your fast, but it's best to avoid it during your fasting period.

Can I drink flavored coffee?

Drinking coffee made with flavored coffee beans is sometimes okay while fasting. However, choosing a coffee that doesn't have added sugar or other sweeteners is essential.

Other Fasting Friendly Drinks

Here are some other drinks you can enjoy while fasting:

Water

Drinking plenty of water is essential for overall health and can also help to keep you hydrated during your fast.

Sparkling Water

Drinking sparkling water is a great way to stay hydrated and avoid feeling thirsty during your fast. Just be sure to choose sparkling water without added sugar or other sweeteners.

Tea

Tea is an excellent choice for fasting as it contains zero calories. Just be sure to avoid adding milk or sugar to your tea. Black tea, green tea, and herbal tea are all calorie-free and can help to boost your metabolism.

Unsweetened Herbal Tea

Drinking herbal tea is a beautiful way to stay hydrated during your fast. Just be sure to choose an herbal tea that doesn't have added sugar or other sweeteners.

Chapter Fifteen Summary:

Now that we have taken this deep dive into coffee and fasting, let's recap what we learned.

1. Black coffee is the best coffee to drink while intermittent fasting, as it doesn't break your fast.
2. Adding dairy or plant-based milk to your coffee can break your fast.
3. Bulletproof coffee will also break your fast.
4. Drinking flavored coffee is sometimes okay while fasting, but be sure to choose a coffee without added sugar or other sweeteners.
5. Other great choices for fasting include water, sparkling water, tea, and unsweetened herbal tea.

So there you have it, everything you need to know about coffee and fasting. Now go forth and enjoy your cup of joe without breaking your fast!

The next chapter focuses on staying inspired throughout your fasting journey. Join us as we explore the best ways to stay motivated, even when fasting gets tough. Plus, some motivational quotes about intermittent fasting to get you inspired!

You can find all of the research mentioned in this book in Appendix B: Resources near the end.

How To Stay Motivated While Intermittent Fasting

It's no secret that intermittent fasting can be challenging, especially if you're new to the practice. There will be days when you'll feel hangry (hungry + angry) or just downright cranky. And that's okay! It's normal to have off days when fasting.

The key is to find ways to stay motivated, even when the going gets tough. Here are some tips on how to stay motivated while intermittent fasting:

Tip #1. Set realistic goals.

When starting with intermittent fasting, it's essential to set realistic goals. If you're trying to lose weight, don't expect to see results overnight. It takes time and commitment to see results with any weight loss plan, so be patient.

Or, if you're dealing with health issues, don't expect fasting to be a miracle cure. Instead, focus on how you're feeling. Do you have more energy? Are you sleeping better? What have you noticed since starting to fast?

Tip #2. Find a fasting buddy.

One of the best ways to stay motivated while intermittent fasting is to find a fasting buddy. Having someone to share your journey with can make all the difference. In addition, you can encourage each other on days when you're struggling and celebrate your successes together.

Tip #3. Join an online community.

If you can't find a fasting buddy in real life, consider joining an online community. There are many active forums and Facebook groups dedicated to intermittent fasting. This is a great way to connect with others on the same journey as you. In addition, I would love it if you'd subscribe to my wellness blog, LoriGeurin.com, where I support intermittent fasters and those interested in living healthier lives.

Tip #4. Keep a journal.

Another great way to stay motivated while intermittent fasting is to keep a journal. Journaling can help you track your progress, set goals, and reflect on your journey. Plus, it's a great way to release any built-up frustrations you may be feeling.

Tip #5. Focus on positive benefits.

When you're feeling hungry or just plain annoyed, take a step back and focus on the positive benefits of intermittent fasting. Maybe you're losing weight, sleeping better, or having more energy. Whatever the case may be, remind yourself why you started fasting in the first place. Focusing on everything you have to gain from this journey can help you push through the tough times.

Tip #6. Visualize better health.

See yourself healthy, happy, and thriving. Next, visualize how it will feel to reach your health goals. When you have a clear picture in your mind of what you want to achieve, it's easier to stay motivated and committed to your fasting journey. The power of visualization is real, so don't underestimate it!

Tip #7. Take it one day at a time.

If you're feeling overwhelmed, take a step back and focus on taking things one day at a time. This journey is a marathon, not a sprint. You didn't get to your current state of health overnight, so please don't expect to reverse it in that amount of time, either. On the other hand, small steps lead to big changes, so be patient and consistent with your intermittent fasting practice.

Tip #5. Find an inspiring quote.

If you're ever feeling down or unmotivated, find an inspiring quote to lift your spirits. So many quotes about intermittent fasting and health can help you stay on track. Here are 42 of my favorites!

42 Intermittent Fasting Quotes To Inspire You

1. "Fasting is the single greatest natural healing therapy. It is nature's ancient, universal 'remedy' for many problems." – Elson Haas, M.D.
2. "Everyone who does intermittent fasting talks about it as a lifestyle, not a diet. They come for the weight loss, but stay for the health benefits." – author unknown
3. "I assert that fasting is the most efficient means for correcting any disease." – Adolph Mayer, M.D.
4. "Fasting for many people becomes not only a physical but also an emotional and spiritual process." – Cynthia Thurlow
5. "Fasting and natural diet, though essentially unknown as a therapy, should be the first treatment when someone discovers that he or she has a medical problem." – Joel Fuhrman
6. "The best of all medicines is resting and fasting." – Benjamin Franklin
7. "Fasting for the body is food for the soul." – Saint John Chrysostom
8. "I fast for greater physical and mental efficiency." – Plato
9. "Fasting is not nearly so deadly as feasting." – J. Harold Smith
10. "During a fast, you will find out if it is you that controls your thoughts or if it is your thoughts that control you." – author unknown

11. "Through long years of misinformation, people have been told, 'Breakfast is the most important meal of the day. It gives you the strength, energy, and vitality to do a hard morning's work, either physically or mentally." This is absolutely erroneous! It is not a true scientific fact. When you eat a heavy breakfast, through reflex action you feel full and satisfied, but you do not gain straight. It takes hours for this food to be processed by the digestive system before you can gain any energy or vitality from a big breakfast. Digestion is a most highly complicated process. " – Dr. Paul C. Bragg

12. "You're not going to burn body fat if you're eating." – Dr. Jason Fung

13. "Everyone has a doctor in him or her; we just have to help it in its work. The natural healing force within each one of us is the greatest force in getting well. Our food should be our medicine. Our medicine should be our food. But to eat when you are sick is to feed your sickness." – Hippocrates

14. "Through fasting…I have found perfect health, a new state of existence, a feeling of purity and happiness, something unknown to humans." – Upton Sinclair

15. "Fasting blinds the body in order to open your soul." – Rumi

16. "What if I told you that intermittent fasting was really intermittent eating?" – author unknown

17. "Eat a double whopper, and no one bats an eyelash. Fasting for 16 hours …everyone loses their minds!" – author unknown

18. "Fasting is like spring cleaning for your body." – Jentezen Franklin

19. "Intermittent fasting…the diet for people too lazy to cook a bunch of meals during the day!" – Gin Stephens

20. He who buries his head deep into a nosebag full of food cannot hope to see the invisible world. – Al-Ghazali

21. "He who eats until he is sick must fast until he is well." – English Proverb

22. "In a fast, the body tears down its defective parts and then rebuilds anew when eating is resumed." – Herbert M. Sheldon

23. "The power of when you eat…is stronger than what you eat." – Megan Ramos

24. "Fasting is a calming experience. It is restful…relieves anxiety and tension. It is rarely depressing, and it is often downright exhilarating." – Alan Cott, M.D.

25. "Fasting is a positive, healing thing that I GET to do for my body." – author unknown

26. "Fasting has been practiced throughout history by almost every religion in the world." – author unknown

27. "Intermittent fasting enhances the ability of nerve cells to repair DNA." – Mark Mattson

28. "Your body has two fuel sources: food and stored food. You're switching them when you fast." – Dr. Jason Fung

29. "Fasting is the greatest remedy – the physician within." – Philippus Paracelsus

30. "Hunger is the first element of self-discipline. If you can control what you eat and drink, you can control everything else." – Dr. Umar Faruq Abd-Allah

31. "Fasting is not so much a treatment of illness but a treatment of wellness." – Dr. Jason Fung

32. "Instead of medicine, fast for a day.' – Plutarch

33. "Circadian fasting is a less extreme version of a standard intermittent fast. While IF diets – like 16/8 fast – are very popular, it's not what I would recommend to a first-time faster. Whereas circadian fasting is a great place to begin – it times your meals according to your circadian clock and focuses less on number hours of fasting." – Dr. Amy Shah

34. "You burn fat, rather than sugar, in a fasted state." – Maria Emmerich

35. "A fast is broken with consumption of food or a caloric substance; however, many people who enjoy the benefits of fasting and want to incorporate it as a daily ritual may take a more flexible approach such as a 'fat fast' using coconut oil, MCT oil, grass-fed butter, or cacao butter blended into a warm liquid during their fasted window." – Ali Miller, R.D.

36. "Intermittent fasting is incredibly useful in aiding fat loss, preventing cancer, building muscle, and increasing resilience. Done correctly, it's one of the most painless high-impact ways to live longer."

– Dave Asprey

37. "The price of fasting is zero." – Dr. Jason Fung

38. "On fasting days, picture your ideal body and remember that your body is dipping into its fat reserve for energy and repairing damaged cells. Let that knowledge encourage and support you. Feel your food addiction weakening its hold on you." – David Ortner

39. "Intermittent fasting is a lifestyle. It isn't something that you start today and then ends when you get to some arbitrary "goal weight." Something you start and then stop is a DIET. Intermittent fasting isn't a diet – as I said, it's a lifestyle." – Gin Stephens

40. "Even though autophagy and fasting will promote quick recovery and take care of the inflammation, you need enough sleep, calories, healthy fats, and collagen for adequate healing." – Patricia Cook

41. One of the reasons intermittent fasting can work is that it reconnects you with what hunger feels like. – Chris Mohr

42. "Intermittent fasting definitely and massively increases autophagy. And thanks to our caveman history, it thrived. In

times of little food, lysosomes would race around the body looking for damaged cells, pre-diseased cells, and cells which weren't doing much. It would chop them apart – into their smallest parts – and either burn them for energy or use them to repair other areas. Simply, it would perform miracles without any outside help." – Robert Skinner

Chapter Sixteen Summary:

Intermittent fasting is an excellent tool for achieving better health, but it's not always easy. I hope these tips on how to stay motivated while intermittent fasting helps you on your journey. Remember, take it one day at a time and be patient with yourself. The rewards are worth the effort! You can do this!

You can find all of the research mentioned in this book in Appendix B: Resources near the end.

THANK YOU!

Thank you for downloading and reading this book! I hope you enjoyed reading the book as much as I enjoyed researching and writing it. If you found anything helpful in the book, could you please spare a moment and consider **sharing a quick review** on Amazon? Book reviews are critical to authors, especially when we're starting out. A kind word can make a positive difference, and I would greatly appreciate it if you took the time to leave one for me. Thank you so much!

You may simply scan this QR code to leave a review.

I hope this book has shed light on intermittent fasting and you feel more confident in trying it out for yourself. Remember to start slow, listen to your body, and don't be too hard on yourself if you stumble along the way. Intermittent fasting is not a diet, it's a lifestyle change that can profoundly benefit your health, weight, and energy levels. But like anything worth doing, it takes time and effort to see results. So be patient, stay the course, and enjoy the journey. Who knows, you may just find that intermittent fasting is the key to unlocking a happier, healthier you. Thanks for reading!

Appendix A: Bibliography

Here are a few of the many books that have inspired, informed, and encouraged me on my wellness journey. Some are specific to fasting, and others are related to overall health and well-being. Please know that any mention of a particular eating plan is not an endorsement because, as you know, fasting brings freedom from food restriction. I simply want to share some inspiring reading that has positively impacted my life in hopes that it will do the same for you. I hope you enjoy exploring and reading this list of books as much as I have!

The Complete Guide To Fasting: Heal Your Body Through Intermittent, Alternate-Day, and Extended Fasting

Fast, Feast, Repeat

The Obesity Code: Unlocking The Secrets Of Weight Loss

The Carbohydrate Addict's Diet: The Lifelong Solution To Yo-Yo Dieting

The Wahl's Protocol: A Radical New Way To Treat All Chronic Autoimmune Conditions Using Paleo Principles

The Fast-5 Diet and the Fast-5 Lifestyle: A Little Book About Making Big Changes

Delay, Don't Deny: Living An Intermittent Fasting Lifestyle

Why We Get Fat: And What To Do About It

The Primal Blueprint: Reprogram Your Genes For Effortless Weightloss, Vibrant Health, And Boundless Energy

The China Study: The Most Comprehensive Study Of Nutrition Ever Conducted And The Startling Implications For Diet, Weight Loss, And Long-term Health

What To Say When You Talk To Yourself

Wheat Belly: Lose The Wheat, Lose The Weight, And Find Your Path Back to Health

Boundaries: When To Say Yes, How To Say No To Take Control Of Your Life

Final Thoughts From Lori

Thank you very much for downloading and reading this book! I hope you enjoyed reading it as much as I enjoyed researching and writing it. If you did, could you please spare a minute and consider sharing a quick Amazon review? **You may simply scan the QR code to leave a review.**

Thank you again!

I hope this book opened your eyes to the many benefits of intermittent fasting, such as weight loss, increased brainpower, disease prevention, and even *reversing* disease already done.

IF allows you to pursue a healthier lifestyle in a simple, natural, and affordable way. I hope you feel motivated to make positive changes in your life with all of this book's tools at your disposal.

IF has drastically changed my life for the better, and I'm excited to have this platform to share with you! Because of intermittent fasting, I no longer crave sweets constantly. Consequently, I experience less hunger than before! Additionally, it's helped me lose 25 pounds without feeling like I'm dieting. Plus, cravings don't control me anymore, so I can think more clearly, work more efficiently, and enjoy a sharper memory despite struggling with chronic illness for years.

You, too, can enjoy all of these benefits and more by intermittent fasting! I encourage you to give it a try for yourself. Remember, there is no *one size fits all* fasting approach — so find what works best for you and stick with it.

Thanks again for reading this book. I wish you the best of luck on your intermittent fasting journey!

Appendix B: Resources

Chapter 1: Who This Intermittent Fasting Book Is For

- https://www.cdc.gov/obesity/data/adult.html

Chapter 2: How Intermittent Fasting Reversed My Hypoglycemia

- https://www.ncbi.nlm.nih.gov/pmc/articles/PMC7856758/#:~:text=Results,and%20increasing%20levels%20of%20adiponectin.
- https://pubmed.ncbi.nlm.nih.gov/21484219/#:~:text=Abstract,mononeuropathy%20multiplex%2C%20and%20painful%20radiculoneuritis.
- https://www.ncbi.nlm.nih.gov/pmc/articles/PMC7021351/#:~:text=Intermittent%20fasting%20(IF)%20refers%20to,week%20on%20non%2Dconsecutive%20days.&text=During%20fasting%2C%20caloric%20consumption%20often,to%2025%25%20of%20caloric%20needs.

Chapter 3: So, What Is Intermittent Fasting Anyway?
- https://www.ncbi.nlm.nih.gov/pmc/articles/PMC7021351/#:~:text=Intermittent%20fasting%20(IF)%20refers%20to,week%20on%20non%2Dconsecutive%20days.&text=During%20fasting%2C%20caloric%20consumption%20often,to%2025%25%20of%20caloric%20needs.

Chapter 4: Scientifically Proven Health Benefits Of Intermittent Fasting

- https://www.sciencedirect.com/science/article/abs/pii/S0969996106003251
- https://www.sciencedirect.com/science/article/abs/pii/S193152441400200X
- https://www.ncbi.nlm.nih.gov/pmc/articles/PMC329619/
- https://www.sciencedirect.com/science/article/abs/pii/S193152441400200X
- https://academic.oup.com/geronj/article-abstract/38/1/36/570019
- https://www.ncbi.nlm.nih.gov/pmc/articles/PMC2622429/
- https://www.nature.com/articles/nm.3804
- https://www.sciencedaily.com/releases/2014/06/140614150142.htm
- https://pubmed.ncbi.nlm.nih.gov/22323820/

Chapter 5: Why Intermittent Fasting Is The Simple Way To Lose Weight

- https://www.ncbi.nlm.nih.gov/pmc/articles/PMC7021351/#:~:text=Intermittent%20fasting%20(IF)%20refers%20to,week%20on%20non%2Dconsecutive%20days.&text=During%20fasting%2C%20caloric%20consumption%20often,to%2025%25%20of%20caloric%20needs.
- https://pubmed.ncbi.nlm.nih.gov/2355952/
- https://pubmed.ncbi.nlm.nih.gov/12107252/
- https://pubmed.ncbi.nlm.nih.gov/15640462/

Chapter 6: The 5 Most Popular Intermittent Fasting Methods + Schedules

- https://pubmed.ncbi.nlm.nih.gov/30172870/
- https://www.ncbi.nlm.nih.gov/pmc/articles/PMC329619/
- https://www.ncbi.nlm.nih.gov/pmc/articles/PMC2622429/
- https://www.ncbi.nlm.nih.gov/pmc/articles/PMC2622429/
- https://pubmed.ncbi.nlm.nih.gov/22323820/
- https://www.sciencedaily.com/releases/2014/06/140614150142.htm
- https://www.nature.com/articles/nm.3804
- https://academic.oup.com/geronj/article-abstract/38/1/36/570019

Chapter 7: Who Should NOT Do Intermittent Fasting?

- https://pubmed.ncbi.nlm.nih.gov/34008846/
- https://www.ncbi.nlm.nih.gov/pmc/articles/PMC2850570/

Chapter 8: 9 Key Questions About Intermittent Fasting Answered

- https://pubmed.ncbi.nlm.nih.gov/19538695/
- https://www.ncbi.nlm.nih.gov/pmc/articles/PMC6983467/
- https://pubmed.ncbi.nlm.nih.gov/21410865/
- https://pubmed.ncbi.nlm.nih.gov/23755298/

Chapter 9: 12 Insider Tips For Intermittent Fasting

- https://www.ncbi.nlm.nih.gov/pmc/articles/PMC2908954/

- https://pubmed.ncbi.nlm.nih.gov/30585192/#:~:text=Po
  lyphenols%20are%20the%20major%20active,epicatechin
  %2C%20gallocatechins%20and%20gallocatechin%20gallat
  e.
- https://www.ncbi.nlm.nih.gov/pmc/articles/PMC653690
  4/#:~:text=Current%20recommendations%20for%20phy
  sical%20activity,and%20vigorous%2Dintensity%20aerobic
  %20activity.
- https://www.ncbi.nlm.nih.gov/pmc/articles/PMC443454
  6/#:~:text=Adults%20should%20sleep%207%20or,and%
  20increased%20risk%20of%20death.

Chapter 10: Top 7 Myths About Fasting Debunked

- https://pubmed.ncbi.nlm.nih.gov/35070352/
- https://pubmed.ncbi.nlm.nih.gov/27304506/
- https://www.ncbi.nlm.nih.gov/pmc/articles/PMC883932
  5/
- https://www.ncbi.nlm.nih.gov/pubmed/21410865
- https://pubmed.ncbi.nlm.nih.gov/17413096/
- https://pubmed.ncbi.nlm.nih.gov/9155494/
- https://pubmed.ncbi.nlm.nih.gov/2405717/
- https://www.cambridge.org/core/journals/british-
  journal-of-nutrition/article/div-classtitleacute-effects-on-
  metabolism-and-appetite-profile-of-one-meal-difference-
  in-the-lower-range-of-meal-
  frequencydiv/4AE8C3FC32CE7E456B9606F1AF963E76
- https://www.sciencedirect.com/science/article/abs/pii/S
  0195666399902659

Chapter 11: What Is OMAD, And Is It Right For You?

- https://pubmed.ncbi.nlm.nih.gov/35087416/

- https://www.ncbi.nlm.nih.gov/pmc/articles/PMC5394735/
- https://www.ncbi.nlm.nih.gov/pmc/articles/PMC2645638/

Chapter 13: A Guide to Fasting and Fitness at Any Age

- https://pubmed.ncbi.nlm.nih.gov/32781538/
- https://jissn.biomedcentral.com/articles/10.1186/1550-2783-11-S1-P25
- https://pubmed.ncbi.nlm.nih.gov/26438184/
- https://www.sciencedaily.com/releases/2011/04/110403090259.htm
- https://pubmed.ncbi.nlm.nih.gov/35070352/#:~:text=These%20benefits%20include%20metabolic%20shifts,and%20treatment%20of%20chronic%20disease.

Chapter 14: Insider's Guide to Fasting and Food

- https://pubmed.ncbi.nlm.nih.gov/19335713/#:~:text=Individuals%20with%20high%20intakes%20of,pressure%20and%20serum%20cholesterol%20levels.
- https://www.ncbi.nlm.nih.gov/pmc/articles/PMC8618064/
- https://pubmed.ncbi.nlm.nih.gov/28945458/#:~:text=As%20a%20result%2C%20fermented%20foods,fermented%20foods%20and%20health%20benefits.
- https://pubmed.ncbi.nlm.nih.gov/29263222/#:~:text=Conclusions%3A%20Consumption%20of%20approximately%201,slow%20cognitive%20decline%20with%20aging.
- https://pubmed.ncbi.nlm.nih.gov/28854932/
- https://pubmed.ncbi.nlm.nih.gov/25757894/#:~:text=St

udies%20have%20demonstrated%20that%20higher,term
%20improvements%20in%20bone%20health.

- https://pubmed.ncbi.nlm.nih.gov/30651162/

Chapter 15: Does Coffee Break a Fast?

- https://pubmed.ncbi.nlm.nih.gov/7369170/
- https://pubmed.ncbi.nlm.nih.gov/24769862/#:~:text=Al
together%2C%20these%20results%20indicate%20that,pro
mote%20health%20by%20stimulating%20autophagy.
- https://pubmed.ncbi.nlm.nih.gov/28177691/
- https://pubmed.ncbi.nlm.nih.gov/25636220/

Chapter 16: How To Stay Motivated While Intermittent Fasting

- https://www.ncbi.nlm.nih.gov/pmc/articles/PMC6796622
9/
- https://www.ncbi.nlm.nih.gov/pmc/articles/PMC3830620
/
- https://pubmed.ncbi.nlm.nih.gov/24124985/
- https://www.ncbi.nlm.nih.gov/pmc/articles/PMC6224443
9/

About the Author

Lori is the founder of a leading health and wellness blog, LoriGeurin.com, which has encouraged thousands of readers. After resigning from her teaching job in 2015 because of a debilitating illness caused by untreated Lyme disease, she set out to help others find optimum health. Because of her love for people and her passion for helping others thrive, she became a Certified Holistic Wellness and Life Coach. A life-long nutrition nerd, Lori enjoys researching wellness topics and sharing the latest findings with her amazing readers. She especially loves sharing how intermittent fasting has helped her overcome many health challenges. For example, the intermittent fasting lifestyle cured her reactive hypoglycemia and significantly improved her chronic pain and inflammation.

Lori lives with her husband, David, a school Superintendent, and is a Mom to 4 amazing kids. She earned Bachelor's degrees in Elementary Education, Early Childhood, and Special Education and was studying for her Master's Degree in Autism before her life changed drastically due to untreated Lyme disease. When she's not working with clients, freelance writing, or blogging about fasting and health, she loves the beach, books, sunsets, concerts, and spending time with her family.

Connect With Lori

Wellness Blog—LoriGeurin.com
Pinterest — @LoriGeurin
Facebook — @LoriGeurinBlog
Twitter — @LoriGeurin
Instagram — @LoriGeurin
LinkedIn — @LoriGeurin
Bloglovin — @LoriGeurin
TikTok — @WellnessLori
Etsy Shop — Thrive Berry (etsy.com/shop/thriveberry)
Email — wellnessforlife@lorigeurin.com